Table of Contents

1 Chapter 1: Introduction to Tissue Regeneration . . . 3

1.1 Regeneration Fundamentals 6

1.2 Challenges in Tissue Repair 10

2 Chapter 2: Growth Factor Applications 15

2.1 Growth Factors in Regrowth 18

2.2 Delivery System Innovations 22

2.3 Clinical Trial Outcomes 25

3 Chapter 3: Scaffolding and Biomaterials 31

3.1 Scaffold Design Principles 35

3.2 Biomaterial Selection 38

3.3 Cell-Scaffold Interactions 42

3.4 Applications of Scaffolds 46

3.5 Advancements in 3D Printing 49

4 Chapter 4: Cellular Therapies 53

4.1 Stem Cells in Tissue Repair 57

4.2 Immune Modulation for Healing 60

5 Chapter 5: Environmental Influences 65

5.1 Impact of Oxygen Tension 68

5.2 Role of Mechanical Stimuli 71

5.3 Effects of Inflammation 75

6 Chapter 6: Advanced Regrowth Strategies 79
6.1 Gene Therapy Approaches 82
6.2 Microfluidic Devices in Tissue Eng 85
6.3 Combining Therapies for Success 89

7 Chapter 7: Future Directions and Challenges 93
7.1 Personalized Regrowth Strategies 97
7.2 Ethical Considerations 100
7.3 Moving Towards Clinical Translation 103

1 Chapter 1: Introduction to Tissue Regeneration

Regeneration, at its core, is the body's innate ability to repair or replace damaged tissues, effectively restoring function. This complex process isn't just about patching things up; it's about rebuilding, recreating, and revitalizing. Think of a salamander regrowing its limb, a remarkable feat of nature. While human regeneration isn't quite as dramatic, our bodies possess a surprising capacity for self-repair, albeit often limited and imperfect. To truly understand it, we must look beyond simply closing wounds and consider the cellular and molecular mechanisms orchestrating this intricate dance of regrowth.

The fundamentals lie in understanding the difference between repair and true regeneration. Repair often results in scar tissue, a fibrous patch that restores structural integrity but lacks the original tissue's specialized function. Imagine a deep cut on your skin - it heals, but a scar remains, lacking hair follicles or sweat glands. True regeneration, on the other hand, aims to recreate the original tissue structure and function, essentially erasing the damage. This is where the real challenge lies, as our bodies are more inclined toward repair than complete regeneration. We see varying degrees of regenerative capacity across different tissues. The liver, for instance, possesses a remarkable ability to regenerate after partial removal, while heart tissue has very limited regenerative capabilities. Understanding these inherent differences is crucial for developing targeted therapies.

Diving deeper, the mechanisms driving regrowth are multifaceted, involving a complex interplay of cells, growth factors, and the extracellular matrix (ECM). Cells, specifically stem cells and progenitor cells, are the building blocks of new tissue. These cells can differentiate into specialized cell types, replacing damaged or lost cells. Growth factors act as messengers, signaling cells to proliferate, migrate, and differentiate. Think of them as tiny conductors, guiding the cellular orchestra. The ECM, a structural network surrounding cells, provides support and influences cell behavior. Its composition and organization play a vital role in guiding tissue regeneration. The extracellular matrix and cells interact each other providing the building blocks for tissue regeneration.

Several challenges hinder successful tissue repair, and conquering these is vital for advancing regenerative medicine. Inflammation, a natural response to injury, can often become chronic and detrimental, impeding the healing process. Uncontrolled inflammation can damage surrounding tissues and prevent proper regeneration. Scarring, as previously mentioned, is a common outcome of repair, resulting in functional limitations. Preventing excessive scar formation is a major goal in regenerative medicine. Limited vascularization, or the formation of new blood vessels, can restrict oxygen and nutrient supply to the injured tissue, hindering regeneration. New tissues need a steady supply of blood to thrive. Overcoming these challenges requires innovative strategies that address the underlying causes and promote a regenerative environment.

Inflammation needs to be controlled to maximize success of the healing process. Furthermore, scarring, a common outcome, can restrict functions. Similarly, limited vascularization can restrict oxygen supply, which will hinder regeneration and lead to unwanted cell death. Thus, we can overcome these limits with innovative strategies and promote a regenerative environment. Understanding the fundamentals of regeneration and the challenges it faces is essential for developing effective therapies and pushing the boundaries of what's possible in medicine.

The process is a complex dance of cellular and molecular events, orchestrated to restore tissue integrity and function. However, it's not always a smooth and efficient process. Several challenges can impede successful tissue repair. One of the primary hurdles is inflammation, the body's natural response to injury. While acute inflammation is essential for initiating the healing process, chronic or excessive inflammation can be detrimental, leading to tissue damage and scarring. Controlling inflammation is therefore crucial for promoting regeneration.

Another significant challenge is scarring, the formation of fibrous connective tissue that replaces damaged tissue. While scar tissue provides structural support, it often lacks the specialized function of the original tissue. For instance, scar tissue in the heart can impair its ability to contract and pump blood effectively. Preventing or minimizing scar formation is a major goal in regenerative medicine.

Vascularization, the formation of new blood vessels, is essential for delivering oxygen and nutrients to regenerating tissues. However, in many cases, vascularization is limited, hindering the healing process. Stimulating angiogenesis, the formation of new blood vessels, is therefore a key strategy for promoting tissue regeneration.

The extracellular matrix (ECM), a complex network of proteins and other molecules that surrounds cells, plays a crucial role in tissue regeneration. The ECM provides structural support, regulates cell behavior, and influences tissue development. However, in injured tissues, the ECM can become damaged or degraded, impairing its ability to support regeneration. Restoring or remodeling the ECM is therefore an important aspect of tissue engineering. Moreover, the aged and diseased patient poses unique challenges to tissue regeneration. As we age, our regenerative capacity declines, and age-related conditions such as diabetes and cardiovascular disease can further impair tissue repair. Developing regenerative therapies that are effective in these patient populations is a major challenge.

From a broader perspective, the complexity of tissue regeneration highlights the need for interdisciplinary approaches that integrate biology, engineering, and medicine. Regenerative medicine is not just about repairing damaged tissues; it's about understanding the fundamental processes that govern tissue regeneration and harnessing these processes to develop new therapies. By addressing the challenges and embracing interdisciplinary approaches, we can unlock the full potential of tissue regeneration and improve the lives of patients with a wide range of injuries and diseases. The journey towards effective tissue regeneration is challenging but is brimming with innovative breakthroughs.

1.1 Regeneration Fundamentals

Regeneration isn't simply about patching things up; it's about rebuilding, restructuring, and restoring function to damaged tissues. Consider the humble salamander, capable of regrowing entire limbs, a stark contrast to our limited regenerative capabilities. Understanding why this difference exists is fundamental to our exploration. Our bodies are programmed to prioritize survival, and often, scar tissue formation is the quickest, most efficient route to closure, even if it means sacrificing function. But what if we could reprogram our tissues, nudging them away from scar formation and towards true regeneration? That is the challenge we are looking to tackle.

The first step in understanding regeneration is to appreciate the difference between regeneration and repair. Repair, the body's default response to injury, results in the formation of scar tissue, a dense, collagen-rich matrix that provides structural support but lacks the specialized functions of the original tissue. Think of a skin wound that heals with a scar - the skin is intact, but it may lack hair follicles, sweat glands, and the same elasticity as the surrounding tissue. Regeneration, on the other hand, involves the complete restoration of tissue structure and function, essentially creating a new version of the original tissue. The liver, for example, possesses a remarkable capacity for regeneration, capable of regrowing substantial portions of itself after injury, maintaining its vital metabolic functions. This distinction highlights the critical role of cellular processes that guide proper tissue reconstruction.

Several key cellular and molecular players are involved in the regenerative process. These include stem cells, growth factors, and the extracellular matrix (ECM). Stem cells are undifferentiated cells with the potential to differentiate into various specialized cell types, providing the building blocks for new tissue. Growth factors are signaling molecules that stimulate cell proliferation, differentiation, and migration, orchestrating the regenerative response. The ECM, a complex network of proteins and carbohydrates surrounding cells, provides structural support and regulates cell behavior, influencing tissue organization and function. All of these come together to drive or stifle a proper healing response.

The process begins with an injury, triggering an inflammatory response. While inflammation is often viewed negatively, it is a crucial initial step in regeneration, clearing debris and recruiting immune cells to the site of injury. These immune cells release growth factors and cytokines that stimulate the proliferation and migration of stem cells and other cells involved in tissue regeneration. A carefully orchestrated immune response is essential; excessive or prolonged inflammation can hinder regeneration and promote scar formation. Consider the differences in how a clean surgical incision heals compared to a deep burn. The burn often results in significant scarring due to the prolonged and intense inflammatory response.

Now, what dictates whether a tissue repairs or regenerates? Several factors come into play, including the type of tissue, the extent of injury, and the local microenvironment. Tissues with a high turnover rate, such as skin and blood, tend to have a greater regenerative capacity than tissues with a low turnover rate, such as cartilage and nerves. The extent of injury also plays a crucial role; small injuries are more likely to regenerate than large injuries, where the body may prioritize rapid closure over complete restoration. The local microenvironment, including the presence of growth factors, ECM components, and inflammatory signals, significantly influences cell behavior and the regenerative outcome.

Unfortunately, our bodies aren't naturally adept at regenerating most tissues. Several obstacles stand in the way, preventing us from fully harnessing our regenerative potential. One major hurdle is the formation of scar tissue, which physically blocks cell migration and inhibits tissue remodeling. Another challenge is the limited availability of stem cells in some tissues, hindering their ability to regenerate. Furthermore, the lack of appropriate growth factor signaling and ECM support can prevent cells from differentiating and organizing into functional tissue. Overcoming these obstacles requires a multifaceted approach, combining strategies to minimize scar formation, enhance stem cell recruitment, and optimize the local microenvironment.

Let's consider a practical example: bone regeneration. When a bone fracture occurs, the body initiates a complex cascade of events aimed at repairing the break. Initially, a blood clot forms at the fracture site, followed by inflammation and the recruitment of immune cells. These cells release growth factors that stimulate the proliferation and differentiation of bone-forming cells, called osteoblasts. The osteoblasts then begin to deposit new bone matrix, gradually bridging the gap between the fractured ends. However, if the fracture is large or unstable, the healing process can be impaired, leading to delayed union or non-union. In such cases, interventions such as bone grafting or the application of growth factors may be necessary to stimulate bone regeneration.

To truly understand regeneration, you must grasp its intricate complexity and the multitude of factors that influence its success. By delving into the cellular and molecular mechanisms driving regeneration, identifying the obstacles that hinder it, and exploring innovative strategies to overcome these hurdles, we can pave the way for new therapies that promote tissue regeneration and improve patient outcomes. Think of the possibilities: regenerating damaged hearts after a heart attack, repairing spinal cord injuries to restore mobility, or even regrowing limbs lost to trauma or disease. While these goals may seem ambitious, they are within reach if we continue to unravel the mysteries of regeneration and translate our knowledge into effective clinical therapies. The future of medicine lies in harnessing our own bodies' innate ability to heal and regenerate, leading to a healthier, more resilient future for all.

1.2 Challenges in Tissue Repair

Healing isn't always a straightforward process. While the body possesses an incredible capacity for self-repair, various challenges can significantly hinder the effective regeneration of damaged tissues, sometimes leading to incomplete recovery or chronic conditions. Understanding these obstacles is crucial for developing targeted strategies to overcome them and promote successful healing.

One of the most significant hurdles is the intricate inflammatory response that follows tissue injury. While inflammation is essential for clearing debris and initiating the healing cascade, prolonged or excessive inflammation can be detrimental. Chronic inflammation can damage surrounding tissues, disrupt cellular processes, and prevent the deposition of new extracellular matrix, ultimately leading to scar formation rather than functional tissue regeneration. For instance, in chronic wounds like diabetic ulcers, persistent inflammation driven by factors such as bacterial infection and impaired immune function can stall the healing process indefinitely. Managing the inflammatory response effectively, through interventions like anti-inflammatory drugs or targeted therapies that modulate immune cell activity, is often necessary to create a regenerative environment.

Another significant challenge is the limited regenerative capacity of certain tissues. Some tissues, like skin and liver, possess a remarkable ability to regenerate, while others, such as cardiac muscle and neural tissue, have very limited regenerative potential. This disparity is largely due to differences in the abundance and activity of resident stem cells and the presence of inhibitory signals that prevent cell proliferation and differentiation. In the case of myocardial infarction, for example, damaged heart muscle is typically replaced by scar tissue, which lacks the contractile properties of healthy tissue, leading to impaired cardiac function. Strategies aimed at stimulating endogenous stem cells or delivering exogenous stem cells to the injured tissue hold promise for enhancing regeneration in these tissues, but significant challenges remain in controlling stem cell fate and ensuring their integration into the surrounding tissue.

Furthermore, inadequate vascularization poses a major obstacle to tissue regeneration. Blood vessels are essential for delivering oxygen, nutrients, and growth factors to the injured tissue, as well as removing metabolic waste products. Without sufficient blood supply, cells cannot survive and function properly, and the healing process is severely compromised. This is particularly problematic in large tissue defects or in tissues with poor intrinsic vascularity, such as cartilage. Promoting angiogenesis, the formation of new blood vessels, is therefore a critical goal in tissue engineering and regenerative medicine. This can be achieved through the delivery of angiogenic growth factors, the use of pro-angiogenic biomaterials, or the application of mechanical stimuli that promote vessel growth.

The formation of scar tissue, also known as fibrosis, represents another major challenge. Scarring is the body's natural response to injury when tissue damage is extensive, but it often results in impaired function and aesthetics. Scar tissue is characterized by excessive deposition of collagen, which creates a dense, disorganized matrix that lacks the elasticity and structural integrity of native tissue. In organs like the liver and lungs, fibrosis can lead to organ failure. Preventing or reversing scar formation is a major focus of regenerative medicine research. Strategies include inhibiting the activity of fibrogenic cells, such as myofibroblasts, using antifibrotic drugs, and promoting the degradation of excess collagen through the use of enzymes or biomaterials that stimulate matrix remodeling.

Additionally, the presence of infection can severely impede tissue regeneration. Bacteria, viruses, or fungi can contaminate the wound site, triggering an inflammatory response and damaging surrounding tissues. Infections can also disrupt cellular processes essential for healing, such as cell proliferation, migration, and matrix deposition. Preventing infection through proper wound care and the use of antimicrobial agents is crucial for creating a regenerative environment. In cases of chronic infection, more aggressive interventions, such as surgical debridement and systemic antibiotics, may be necessary.

Age also plays a significant role in tissue regeneration. As we age, our bodies' regenerative capacity declines, and the healing process becomes slower and less efficient. This is due to a variety of factors, including a decrease in the number and activity of stem cells, reduced growth factor production, and impaired immune function. In older individuals, even minor injuries can take longer to heal and may result in more significant scarring. Developing strategies to counteract the age-related decline in regenerative capacity, such as stem cell therapies or interventions that boost growth factor production, is a major area of research.

Finally, the complexity of tissue architecture presents a significant challenge for engineering functional tissues. Tissues are not simply collections of cells; they are highly organized structures with intricate arrangements of cells, extracellular matrix, and blood vessels. Recreating this complex architecture in vitro is a major hurdle in tissue engineering. Advancements in 3D printing and other biofabrication techniques are helping to overcome this challenge by allowing for the precise spatial arrangement of cells and biomaterials, but further research is needed to fully replicate the intricate organization of native tissues.

Overcoming the challenges in tissue repair requires a multidisciplinary approach that integrates knowledge from biology, engineering, and medicine. By understanding the factors that impede regeneration and developing targeted strategies to address them, we can unlock the body's full regenerative potential and improve outcomes for patients with tissue damage and disease. This proactive and innovative approach promises to revolutionize how we approach healing and tissue restoration in the future, offering hope for more complete and functional recoveries.

2 Chapter 2: Growth Factor Applications

Growth factors are the conductors of the cellular orchestra that drives tissue regeneration. They aren't just mere ingredients in the recipe for regrowth; they are the signaling molecules that instruct cells on when to divide, migrate, differentiate, and synthesize extracellular matrix. Understanding their specific roles and how to effectively deliver them is paramount to successful tissue engineering. We must shift our mindset from simply applying growth factors to strategically orchestrating their actions for optimal outcomes in the face of trauma and chronic disease.

One of the first hurdles to overcome is the inherent instability of many growth factors. These delicate proteins are susceptible to degradation by enzymes, changes in pH, and temperature fluctuations within the body. This necessitates the development of delivery systems that can protect them from these harsh conditions, ensuring they reach the target cells in an active form. Think of it like this: you wouldn't ship a precious antique without carefully wrapping it in protective materials; the same principle applies to growth factors. Several strategies have emerged, each with its own advantages and limitations. Microencapsulation, for example, involves encapsulating growth factors within tiny spheres made of biodegradable polymers. This protects them from degradation and allows for sustained release over time. Another approach involves conjugating growth factors to larger molecules, such as heparin or collagen, which can enhance their stability and prolong their residence time at the injury site. These modifications may enhance the overall repair mechanism by acting as a physical scaffold for cells to grow into.

The choice of delivery system depends heavily on the specific growth factor being used and the tissue being targeted. For instance, delivering bone morphogenetic protein-2 (BMP-2) to a bone fracture site requires a different strategy than delivering epidermal growth factor (EGF) to a skin wound. In the former case, a slow-releasing scaffold made of calcium phosphate may be ideal, while in the latter, a hydrogel that can conform to the wound bed and provide a moist environment may be more appropriate. The location of repair is vital to understand when choosing the optimal approach. Beyond simply protecting growth factors, we also need to consider how to deliver them in a targeted manner. Traditional methods, such as direct injection, can lead to widespread distribution of the growth factor throughout the body, potentially causing unwanted side effects. To overcome this, researchers are developing sophisticated delivery systems that can be directed to specific cells or tissues. One promising approach involves using nanoparticles that are coated with antibodies or other targeting molecules that bind to receptors on the surface of target cells. These nanoparticles can then deliver their cargo of growth factors directly to the cells that need them most.

Clinical trials have provided valuable insights into the potential and limitations of growth factor-based therapies. While some trials have shown remarkable success, others have yielded disappointing results. It's important to carefully examine the factors that contribute to these discrepancies. One major factor is the variability in patient populations. Patients with underlying health conditions, such as diabetes or vascular disease, may have impaired healing responses that limit the effectiveness of growth factors. The severity of the injury and the timing of growth factor administration are also critical factors. Growth factors may be more effective when applied early in the healing process, before inflammation becomes excessive and scar tissue begins to form. It is pivotal to remember that a good approach to accelerate the healing of a chronic wound may be less effective in case of acute injury.

Another important consideration is the choice of outcome measures in clinical trials. Traditionally, clinical trials have focused on measuring macroscopic outcomes, such as wound closure or bone fracture healing. However, these measures may not fully capture the complex cellular and molecular events that are driving tissue regeneration. To gain a more complete understanding of the efficacy of growth factors, it's essential to incorporate more sensitive and specific outcome measures, such as gene expression analysis, protein profiling, and histological analysis. Additionally, while some growth factors have shown promise in preclinical studies, their clinical translation has been hindered by safety concerns. For example, high doses of certain growth factors have been associated with increased risk of cancer. Therefore, it's crucial to carefully evaluate the safety profile of each growth factor before it is used in clinical trials.

To maximize the potential of growth factor-based therapies, we need to move beyond simply delivering growth factors in isolation. We need to develop combination therapies that integrate growth factors with other regenerative medicine strategies, such as cell therapy and biomaterial scaffolds. The growth factors act as signaling molecules, while the scaffold provides a physical support structure and the cells provide the building blocks for new tissue formation. By combining these elements, we can create a synergistic effect that promotes more robust and complete tissue regeneration. The symphony orchestra is led by the growth factors; they alone cannot play the music.

Furthermore, the future of growth factor applications lies in personalized medicine. Just as each patient's genetic makeup is unique, so too is their response to growth factors. By analyzing a patient's genetic profile and other clinical data, we can identify individuals who are most likely to benefit from a particular growth factor therapy and tailor the treatment accordingly. For instance, we might identify patients who have a genetic predisposition to impaired growth factor signaling and then select a growth factor that is less susceptible to this impairment. The correct identification of the patient's needs plays a vital role in a proper recovery. This personalized approach has the potential to significantly improve the efficacy of growth factor-based therapies and reduce the risk of adverse effects. Therefore, it is paramount to avoid thinking about a single treatment option, and carefully consider all available elements, by choosing the optimal plan and creating a unique, effective, and personalized pathway.

2.1 Growth Factors in Regrowth

Growth factors are the conductors of the cellular orchestra, orchestrating the complex symphony of events required for tissue regrowth. These naturally occurring proteins act as signaling molecules, binding to receptors on cell surfaces and triggering intracellular pathways that influence cell proliferation, differentiation, migration, and survival. Understanding their specific roles and how to harness their power is crucial for anyone venturing into the realm of regenerative medicine. Each growth factor boasts a unique repertoire, and selecting the right combination, delivered at the appropriate time and concentration, can significantly enhance the healing process. Let's look at some of them.

Transforming Growth Factor Beta (TGF-) stands as a pivotal player in tissue repair, known for its multifaceted roles. While sometimes associated with fibrosis and scarring, TGF- isoforms, particularly TGF-1, TGF-2, and TGF-3, are essential for initiating wound healing cascades. They stimulate the production of extracellular matrix (ECM) components like collagen, fibronectin, and proteoglycans, which provide structural support for newly forming tissue. Further, TGF- influences cellular differentiation, guiding fibroblasts towards becoming myofibroblasts, crucial for wound contraction. The concentration and timing of TGF- activity are critical; dysregulation can lead to excessive ECM deposition and scar formation, hence why controlled delivery is so important.

Next is Platelet-Derived Growth Factor (PDGF). Released from platelets during the initial stages of injury, PDGF serves as a potent chemoattractant for immune cells, fibroblasts, and smooth muscle cells. PDGF stimulates cell proliferation and angiogenesis, the formation of new blood vessels. By recruiting cells to the site of injury and stimulating their growth, PDGF helps lay the foundation for tissue regeneration. However, like TGF-, excessive PDGF activity can contribute to fibrosis. Therefore, its application needs to be carefully calibrated to optimize its regenerative potential.

Vascular Endothelial Growth Factor (VEGF) is indispensable for angiogenesis, the formation of new blood vessels, a process crucial for tissue survival and regeneration. Without an adequate blood supply, cells cannot receive the nutrients and oxygen they need to thrive.

VEGF stimulates endothelial cell proliferation, migration, and tube formation, leading to the development of a functional microvasculature within the regenerating tissue. Different isoforms of VEGF exist, each with slightly different properties and affinities for specific receptors. Understanding these nuances allows for targeted delivery and optimized angiogenic responses.

Fibroblast Growth Factors (FGFs) constitute a family of growth factors with diverse roles in tissue development, maintenance, and repair. FGFs influence cell proliferation, differentiation, migration, and survival across a wide range of tissues. FGF-2, in particular, is known for its potent angiogenic and mitogenic properties, promoting both blood vessel formation and cell division. Others, like FGF-7 (also known as keratinocyte growth factor or KGF), specifically target epithelial cells, stimulating their proliferation and migration, critical for wound closure and skin regeneration.

Epidermal Growth Factor (EGF) primarily targets epithelial cells, stimulating their proliferation and differentiation. It is vital for skin regeneration, wound closure, and the formation of new epithelial linings in various organs. EGF activates intracellular signaling pathways that promote cell survival and inhibit apoptosis (programmed cell death). In addition, EGF plays a role in modulating inflammation and stimulating ECM production. Its application can accelerate wound healing, particularly in chronic wounds where epithelialization is impaired.

Delivering these growth factors effectively is as critical as selecting the right ones. Traditional methods of delivery, such as simple injections, often result in rapid degradation and limited bioavailability. Therefore, researchers are constantly developing innovative delivery systems to improve growth factor stability, prolong their release, and target their delivery to specific cells and tissues.

One promising approach involves using biomaterial scaffolds as growth factor carriers. These scaffolds can be designed to release growth factors in a controlled manner over time, providing sustained stimulation to the regenerating tissue. The choice of biomaterial and the method of incorporating growth factors into the scaffold can significantly impact the release kinetics. For instance, growth factors can be physically entrapped within the scaffold matrix or chemically conjugated to the biomaterial.

Another approach is through the use of nanoparticles or microparticles. These particles can encapsulate growth factors and protect them from degradation, while also allowing for targeted delivery to specific cell types. The size, shape, and surface properties of the particles can be tailored to optimize their uptake by cells and their distribution within the tissue. Furthermore, particles can be engineered to release growth factors in response to specific stimuli, such as changes in pH or temperature.

Gene therapy offers another promising avenue for growth factor delivery. By introducing genes encoding growth factors directly into cells, it is possible to achieve sustained and localized production of these proteins. Viral vectors, such as adeno-associated viruses (AAVs), are commonly used to deliver genes to target cells. However, non-viral methods, such as plasmid DNA delivery, are also being explored to reduce the risk of immune responses.

The future of growth factor-based therapies lies in personalized approaches that consider individual patient characteristics and the specific needs of the tissue being regenerated. Factors such as age, genetics, and the presence of comorbidities can all influence the response to growth factors. By understanding these variables and tailoring growth factor delivery accordingly, it may be possible to achieve more predictable and effective outcomes in tissue regeneration. The integration of advanced technologies, such as microfluidic devices and 3D bioprinting, will further enhance the precision and control over growth factor delivery, paving the way for the development of novel regenerative medicine strategies.

Navigating the world of growth factors is no simple task, but understanding these key players and their delivery methods unlocks a powerful toolkit for tissue regrowth. As you delve deeper into this field, remember that the key is to tailor your approach, selecting the right combination of growth factors and delivery systems to meet the specific needs of each unique healing challenge.

2.2 Delivery System Innovations

Targeted release systems represent a leap forward in delivering growth factors precisely where and when they're needed, significantly improving the therapeutic outcome. Instead of flooding the entire system with these potent molecules, which can lead to off-target effects and systemic complications, these systems allow for localized and controlled delivery, maximizing their impact on the damaged tissue while minimizing unwanted side effects. For instance, think of a scenario where you need to repair a small bone fracture. Simply injecting a growth factor might stimulate bone growth in surrounding areas, leading to bone spurs or other undesirable outcomes. A targeted delivery system, however, would ensure that the growth factor is released only at the fracture site, promoting focused healing.

These innovative systems come in various forms, each with its own set of advantages and disadvantages. One popular approach involves encapsulating growth factors within micro or nanoparticles. These particles, typically made from biodegradable polymers, act as protective shells, shielding the growth factors from degradation within the body. The release of the growth factor can be triggered by various stimuli, such as changes in pH, temperature, or enzymatic activity. In the case of an inflamed wound, the slightly acidic environment can trigger the breakdown of the particles, releasing the growth factor precisely where it's needed to stimulate healing. The size and composition of these particles can be carefully tailored to control the rate of release, ensuring a sustained and controlled delivery over time. Another promising strategy involves using hydrogels, which are three-dimensional networks of polymers that can absorb large amounts of water. These hydrogels can be loaded with growth factors and injected into the defect site, providing a scaffold for cell attachment and growth while simultaneously releasing the therapeutic agent. The properties of the hydrogel, such as its stiffness and degradation rate, can be tuned to match the characteristics of the surrounding tissue, creating a more natural and conducive environment for regeneration.

Beyond simple encapsulation, researchers are also exploring more sophisticated delivery mechanisms that can actively target specific cells or tissues. One such approach involves attaching targeting ligands, such as antibodies or peptides, to the surface of the delivery system. These ligands recognize and bind to specific receptors on target cells, ensuring that the growth factor is delivered precisely to the cells that need it most. For example, in the context of nerve regeneration, a delivery system could be functionalized with a ligand that binds to receptors on neurons, directing the growth factor specifically to the damaged nerve cells and promoting their regrowth. This targeted approach not only enhances the efficacy of the therapy but also reduces the risk of off-target effects by minimizing exposure to non-target cells. Furthermore, some delivery systems are designed to respond to external stimuli, such as light or ultrasound. These stimuli can be used to trigger the release of the growth factor on demand, allowing for precise control over the timing and location of delivery.

One of the key challenges in developing these delivery systems is ensuring that the growth factor remains stable and active during the delivery process. Growth factors are often delicate molecules that can be easily degraded by enzymes or other factors in the body. To address this challenge, researchers are exploring various strategies to protect the growth factor, such as encapsulating it in a protective matrix or chemically modifying it to make it more resistant to degradation. Another challenge is achieving a sustained and controlled release of the growth factor over time. An initial burst of growth factor can be detrimental, leading to excessive cell proliferation or other unwanted effects. Ideally, the growth factor should be released gradually over a period of days or weeks, mimicking the natural healing process. To achieve this, researchers are carefully controlling the properties of the delivery system, such as its degradation rate and porosity.

Let's consider the integration of these delivery systems with scaffolding materials; it provides a synergistic effect that can significantly enhance tissue regrowth. By incorporating growth factor-loaded microparticles into a scaffold, you create a microenvironment that is both structurally supportive and biochemically stimulating. The scaffold provides a framework for cells to attach and grow, while the controlled release of growth factors promotes cell proliferation, differentiation, and matrix deposition. The beauty of this approach lies in its ability to mimic the natural healing process, where the body gradually releases growth factors and other signaling molecules to orchestrate tissue repair. Furthermore, the scaffold can protect the growth factors from degradation, extending their therapeutic lifespan. I believe the combination of targeted growth factor delivery with advanced biomaterials represents a powerful strategy for promoting tissue regrowth.

The journey from laboratory bench to bedside is paved with rigorous testing and optimization. Preclinical studies are essential for evaluating the safety and efficacy of these delivery systems in animal models before they can be tested in humans. These studies help to identify potential toxicities and optimize the dosage and delivery regimen. It is equally important to assess the long-term effects of these therapies, ensuring that they do not lead to any adverse outcomes. Finally, clinical trials are needed to confirm the safety and efficacy of these delivery systems in humans. These trials involve carefully designed studies that compare the outcomes of patients treated with the new therapy to those treated with standard treatments.

2.3 Clinical Trial Outcomes

Clinical trial outcomes for growth factor applications in tissue regeneration are a nuanced landscape, filled with both promise and persistent challenges. They represent the culmination of years of research, moving from the controlled environment of the lab to the complex reality of the human body. Early studies, often conducted in vitro or in animal models, established the potential of growth factors to stimulate cell proliferation, migration, and differentiation - the fundamental processes of tissue regrowth. However, translating these successes into consistent and predictable results in human clinical trials has proven to be a significant hurdle. The variability in patient populations, the complexity of wound healing processes, and

the challenges of delivering growth factors effectively all contribute to the mixed bag of outcomes we observe today.
Understanding these outcomes requires a critical evaluation of several key factors. For example, the specific growth factor used is paramount. Different growth factors exert different effects on different cell types and tissues. Bone morphogenetic proteins (BMPs), for instance, have shown remarkable success in promoting bone regeneration, with clinical trials demonstrating their effectiveness in treating non-union fractures. However, their application in soft tissue repair has yielded less consistent results. Similarly, platelet-derived growth factor (PDGF) has shown promise in promoting wound healing in diabetic ulcers, but its efficacy can be highly dependent on the specific formulation and delivery method. The choice of growth factor must be carefully matched to the specific tissue being targeted and the underlying pathophysiology of the injury. Moreover, we need to analyze trial designs, patient populations, and endpoints.
Another critical consideration is the delivery system employed. Growth factors are inherently unstable molecules, prone to degradation and rapid clearance from the injury site. This can limit their therapeutic efficacy and necessitate frequent, high-dose administrations, which can increase the risk of adverse effects. Innovative delivery systems, such as hydrogels, microspheres, and gene therapy vectors, have been developed to address these challenges. Hydrogels, for example, can provide a sustained release of growth factors over time, while microspheres can protect growth factors from degradation and facilitate their targeted delivery to specific cells. Gene therapy vectors can deliver genes encoding growth factors directly to cells, enabling them to produce their own growth factors in situ. Clinical trials evaluating these delivery systems have shown promising results, with improved tissue regeneration and reduced

side effects compared to traditional bolus injections. However, further optimization of these delivery systems is needed to achieve optimal therapeutic outcomes.

The patient population being studied also plays a crucial role in determining clinical trial outcomes. Factors such as age, underlying health conditions, and lifestyle choices can significantly influence the regenerative capacity of tissues and their response to growth factor therapy. For example, patients with diabetes often exhibit impaired wound healing due to compromised blood supply and reduced growth factor signaling. Clinical trials targeting diabetic ulcers have shown that growth factor therapy can improve wound closure rates, but the magnitude of the effect can vary considerably depending on the severity of the diabetes and the presence of other comorbidities. Similarly, older patients may exhibit reduced regenerative capacity due to age-related decline in stem cell activity and growth factor responsiveness. Careful patient selection and stratification are essential to minimize variability and ensure that clinical trials are adequately powered to detect meaningful treatment effects. Considering these parameters can positively affect the results, and improve the lives of patients involved in the trials.

Furthermore, the endpoints used to assess clinical trial outcomes must be carefully chosen to reflect the specific goals of the therapy and the underlying biology of the tissue being regenerated. Traditional endpoints, such as wound closure rate or bone union time, may not always capture the full extent of tissue regeneration. More sophisticated endpoints, such as histological analysis, biomechanical testing, and functional assessments, can provide a more comprehensive evaluation of tissue quality and long-term durability. The use of imaging modalities, such as magnetic resonance imaging (MRI) and computed tomography (CT), can also provide valuable insights into the structural and functional properties of regenerated tissues. It is important to select endpoints that are both clinically relevant and scientifically rigorous to ensure that clinical trial outcomes are meaningful and interpretable.

Despite the challenges, clinical trials of growth factor applications in tissue regeneration have yielded some notable successes. As previously mentioned, BMPs have become a mainstay in the treatment of non-union fractures, significantly reducing the need for bone grafting and improving patient outcomes. PDGF has also shown promise in promoting wound healing in diabetic ulcers, although its efficacy can be variable. Other growth factors, such as transforming growth factor-beta (TGF-) and vascular endothelial growth factor (VEGF), are being actively investigated for their potential to promote soft tissue regeneration and angiogenesis. The results of these trials are eagerly awaited and will help to further define the role of growth factors in regenerative medicine.

Moving forward, several strategies can be employed to improve clinical trial outcomes for growth factor applications. First, a greater emphasis should be placed on preclinical studies to optimize growth factor selection, delivery systems, and treatment protocols. Second, clinical trials should be designed to carefully stratify patients based on their underlying health conditions and regenerative capacity. Third, more sophisticated endpoints should be used to assess the quality and durability of regenerated tissues. Fourth, a greater effort should be made to understand the mechanisms by which growth factors exert their effects in vivo, using techniques such as transcriptomics and proteomics. Finally, greater collaboration between researchers, clinicians, and industry partners is needed to accelerate the translation of promising research findings into clinically viable therapies. By addressing these challenges and embracing these strategies, we can unlock the full potential of growth factors to promote tissue regeneration and improve the lives of patients suffering from a wide range of injuries and diseases.

Finally, it's essential to consider the economic aspects of these therapies. Growth factor-based treatments can be expensive, and cost-effectiveness analyses are crucial for determining their long-term value. These analyses should consider factors such as reduced hospital stays, decreased need for additional surgeries, and improved patient quality of life. Only through a holistic approach that considers both clinical efficacy and economic viability can we ensure that growth factor therapies are accessible and sustainable in the long run.

3 Chapter 3: Scaffolding and Biomaterials

The ideal scaffold acts as a temporary, three-dimensional template that mimics the extracellular matrix (ECM), guiding cellular behavior and facilitating tissue formation. Scaffold design is not a one-size-fits-all approach; rather, it demands careful consideration of the target tissue's specific requirements. This means understanding the tissue's native architecture, mechanical properties, and biological cues. For example, bone scaffolds require high compressive strength and the ability to promote mineralization, while cartilage scaffolds necessitate elasticity and support for chondrocyte differentiation. A critical aspect is porosity, which dictates cell infiltration, nutrient transport, and waste removal. Too little porosity restricts cell migration and vascularization, leading to necrosis. Too much porosity, on the other hand, compromises mechanical integrity. Therefore, optimizing pore size and interconnectivity is paramount. Beyond porosity, scaffold surface topography plays a significant role. Micro\item and nano-scale features can influence cell adhesion, proliferation, and differentiation. For instance, rougher surfaces tend to enhance osteoblast adhesion and bone formation, while smoother surfaces may be preferred for soft tissue applications. Chemical modifications, such as incorporating cell-adhesive peptides like RGD, can further enhance cell-scaffold interactions. Finally, the degradation rate of the scaffold must be carefully controlled to match the rate of new tissue formation. If the scaffold degrades too quickly, it loses its mechanical support before the tissue has fully developed. If it degrades too slowly, it can hinder tissue remodeling and integration.

Biomaterial selection is inextricably linked to scaffold design. The choice of biomaterial dictates the scaffold's mechanical properties, degradation rate, and biocompatibility. Biomaterials can be broadly classified into natural and synthetic polymers. Natural polymers, such as collagen, gelatin, and alginate, offer inherent biocompatibility and biodegradability, as they are derived from the body's own ECM components. Collagen, for instance, is a major component of skin, bone, and cartilage, making it a popular choice for tissue engineering applications. However, natural polymers often lack the mechanical strength and control over degradation rate offered by synthetic polymers. Synthetic polymers, such as poly(lactic acid) (PLA), poly(glycolic acid) (PGA), and poly(-caprolactone) (PCL), can be precisely tailored to achieve desired mechanical properties and degradation kinetics. PLA, for example, is a rigid polymer with a relatively slow degradation rate, making it suitable for load-bearing applications. PGA, on the other hand, degrades more rapidly and is often used in sutures and temporary implants. PCL offers excellent flexibility and biocompatibility, but its slow degradation rate limits its use in some applications. Hybrid biomaterials, combining natural and synthetic polymers, offer a promising approach to leverage the advantages of both. For example, a composite scaffold of collagen and PCL can provide the biocompatibility of collagen and the mechanical strength and controlled degradation of PCL. In addition to polymers, ceramics and metals are also used in tissue engineering, particularly for bone regeneration. Ceramics, such as hydroxyapatite and tricalcium phosphate, are highly biocompatible and osteoconductive, promoting bone cell attachment and mineralization. Metals, such as titanium and its alloys, offer excellent mechanical strength and corrosion resistance, making them suitable for load-bearing implants.

The success of a scaffold hinges on its ability to interact favorably with cells. Cell-scaffold interactions are complex and multifaceted, involving cell adhesion, migration, proliferation, and differentiation. Cell adhesion is the first critical step, mediated by integrins, transmembrane receptors that bind to ECM proteins. Scaffolds must provide appropriate ligands for integrin binding to facilitate cell attachment. As mentioned earlier, incorporating cell-adhesive peptides like RGD can enhance cell adhesion. Cell migration is essential for cells to populate the scaffold and form a functional tissue. The scaffold's pore size, interconnectivity, and surface topography influence cell migration. Cells prefer to migrate along surfaces with high curvature and optimal pore size. Cell proliferation is necessary to increase cell numbers within the scaffold and form a dense tissue. The scaffold must provide adequate nutrients and growth factors to support cell proliferation. The degradation rate of the scaffold can also influence cell proliferation, as degradation products can sometimes be toxic to cells. Cell differentiation is the process by which cells specialize into specific cell types. The scaffold can influence cell differentiation through mechanical cues, chemical signals, and cell-cell interactions. For example, applying compressive forces to chondrocytes within a scaffold can promote cartilage formation. Incorporating growth factors, such as transforming growth factor-beta (TGF-), can also direct cell differentiation.

Scaffolds find diverse applications across various tissue engineering fields. In bone tissue engineering, scaffolds are used to repair bone fractures, fill bone defects, and regenerate bone lost due to trauma or disease. These scaffolds often incorporate hydroxyapatite or tricalcium phosphate to promote bone mineralization. Cartilage tissue engineering utilizes scaffolds to repair damaged cartilage in joints, such as the knee and hip. These scaffolds typically require elasticity and the ability to support chondrocyte differentiation. Skin tissue engineering employs scaffolds to treat burns, wounds, and skin ulcers. These scaffolds provide a temporary barrier to infection and promote cell migration and tissue regeneration. Nerve tissue engineering focuses on using scaffolds to guide nerve regeneration after injury or disease. These scaffolds often incorporate growth factors and neurotrophic factors to stimulate nerve cell growth and differentiation. Vascular tissue engineering utilizes scaffolds to create artificial blood vessels for bypass surgery or to replace damaged vessels. These scaffolds must be biocompatible, flexible, and able to withstand blood pressure.

Additive manufacturing, commonly known as 3D printing, has revolutionized scaffold fabrication. 3D printing allows for the creation of customized scaffolds with precise architecture, pore size, and interconnectivity. This technology enables the fabrication of scaffolds that closely mimic the native tissue structure, improving cell infiltration, nutrient transport, and tissue regeneration. Several 3D printing techniques are used for scaffold fabrication, including fused deposition modeling (FDM), selective laser sintering (SLS), and bioprinting. FDM involves extruding a molten thermoplastic material through a nozzle to create a 3D structure layer by layer. SLS uses a laser to fuse powdered materials together, creating a solid structure. Bioprinting involves dispensing cells and biomaterials to create a 3D tissue construct. 3D printing offers several advantages over traditional scaffold fabrication methods, including increased design flexibility, reduced manufacturing time, and improved control over scaffold properties. Furthermore, 3D printing enables the incorporation of multiple materials and cell types into a single scaffold, creating complex tissue constructs with enhanced functionality. As 3D printing technology continues to advance, it holds great promise for creating personalized scaffolds for tissue regeneration.

3.1 Scaffold Design Principles

Scaffold design is not just about creating a structure; it's about orchestrating a cellular symphony. To begin, understand that every tissue has its unique needs. Bone, cartilage, skin - each demands a specific architecture and material property from its scaffold. Don't fall into the trap of believing one-size-fits-all. Your first question should always be: What is the native tissue like, and how can I mimic that? This understanding forms the bedrock of intelligent scaffold design.

Now, let's dive into porosity. This is arguably the most critical aspect, influencing everything from cell infiltration to nutrient transport. Think of it as the highway system for cells and essential molecules. Too little porosity, and cells suffocate, unable to penetrate and proliferate. Too much, and the scaffold loses its structural integrity, collapsing before it can support new tissue formation. The optimal pore size isn't a fixed number; it varies depending on the cell type and the tissue you're trying to regenerate. For instance, bone regeneration typically requires larger pores (hundreds of micrometers) to allow for vascularization and bone ingrowth, while softer tissues like skin might benefit from smaller pores that encourage cell attachment and migration. Consider using a gradient porosity, mimicking the natural transition zones found in many tissues. This can guide cell differentiation and tissue organization in a spatially controlled manner.

Mechanical properties are equally crucial. Scaffolds must possess the right stiffness and elasticity to withstand the forces they'll experience within the body. Imagine trying to regenerate cartilage with a scaffold as rigid as bone - the cells would be stressed and unable to differentiate properly. On the other hand, a scaffold that's too soft might deform under load, compromising its structural support and hindering tissue formation. The key is to match the mechanical properties of the native tissue as closely as possible. This often involves incorporating materials with tunable mechanical properties or creating composite scaffolds with varying stiffness in different regions. Furthermore, consider the long-term behavior of the scaffold. Will it degrade too quickly, leaving the newly formed tissue unsupported? Or will it persist for too long, interfering with tissue remodeling? The degradation rate should be carefully matched to the rate of new tissue formation, ensuring that the scaffold provides support when needed but eventually disappears, allowing the newly formed tissue to assume its full functionality.

Surface chemistry is the unsung hero of scaffold design. It's the first point of contact between cells and the scaffold, influencing cell adhesion, proliferation, and differentiation. A hydrophobic surface might repel cells, while a hydrophilic surface can promote cell attachment. Modifying the surface with bioactive molecules, such as peptides or growth factors, can further enhance cell-scaffold interactions. For example, incorporating RGD peptides (a common cell adhesion sequence) can significantly improve cell attachment and spreading on the scaffold surface. Think about functionalizing your scaffold's surface to attract specific cell types or to promote differentiation down a particular lineage. This level of control can dramatically improve the success of your tissue regeneration strategy. I once worked on a project where we used a plasma treatment to modify the surface of a polycaprolactone scaffold, significantly improving its hydrophilicity and cell attachment.

Consider the architecture of your scaffold. Is it a simple, uniform structure, or a complex, three-dimensional network? Modern 3D printing techniques allow for the creation of scaffolds with intricate geometries and precise control over pore size and distribution. This opens up exciting possibilities for mimicking the complex architecture of native tissues. For instance, you could create a scaffold with interconnected pores to facilitate vascularization, or a scaffold with different compartments to guide the differentiation of multiple cell types. Think about the microenvironment that you want to create within the scaffold. Are there specific regions that need to be enriched with nutrients or growth factors? Are there specific gradients that need to be established to guide cell migration? By carefully designing the scaffold architecture, you can create a microenvironment that promotes optimal tissue regeneration.

Finally, remember that the best scaffold is one that is biocompatible and non-toxic. The material you choose should not elicit an adverse immune response or release harmful degradation products. Thoroughly test your scaffold in vitro and in vivo to ensure its safety and efficacy. Choose materials that have a proven track record of biocompatibility and that are easily sterilizable. Consider the long-term effects of the scaffold on the surrounding tissue. Will it cause inflammation or fibrosis? Will it interfere with the normal remodeling process? By carefully considering these factors, you can minimize the risk of adverse events and maximize the chances of successful tissue regeneration.

Effective scaffold design is a balancing act, a careful consideration of multiple factors that all contribute to the final outcome. It requires a deep understanding of tissue biology, materials science, and engineering principles. By approaching scaffold design with a holistic perspective, you can create structures that not only provide physical support but also actively promote tissue regeneration. Don't be afraid to experiment and iterate, learning from both your successes and your failures. The field of tissue engineering is constantly evolving, and there's always room for innovation and improvement. Keep pushing the boundaries of what's possible, and you'll be well on your way to developing the next generation of tissue regeneration tools.

3.2 Biomaterial Selection

Selecting the right biomaterial is a foundational step toward successful tissue regrowth. It's not just about finding a substance that the body won't reject; it's about finding one that actively encourages cells to thrive, differentiate, and rebuild damaged tissue in the face of internal and external stressors. This decision requires a deep dive into material properties, biocompatibility, and the specific demands of the target tissue. This is where the science of material selection becomes an art, melding engineering principles with biological understanding.

The properties of a biomaterial are paramount. We need to think beyond simple biocompatibility, considering aspects like porosity, degradation rate, mechanical strength, and surface chemistry. Porosity, for instance, is crucial for cell infiltration and nutrient transport, but the ideal pore size varies depending on the cell type and tissue being regenerated. A bone scaffold will require larger pores to accommodate osteoblast migration and bone matrix deposition, compared to the dense matrix of a heart valve, where we might prioritize smaller pores to prevent thrombus formation. Similarly, the degradation rate must match the rate of new tissue formation. If the material degrades too quickly, the cells won't have adequate support to form new tissue. Too slow, and the scaffold remains in the body, potentially causing long-term complications or hindering natural tissue remodeling. The mechanical strength is crucial for weight-bearing tissues like bone and cartilage, where the biomaterial must withstand significant stress. Finally, the surface chemistry of a biomaterial is what cells "see" first, and it can significantly influence cell attachment, proliferation, and differentiation.

Biocompatibility encompasses more than just avoiding an outright rejection. It is a spectrum, ranging from inertness to active integration with the host tissue. The ideal biomaterial will not only be non-toxic and non-immunogenic but will also actively promote cell adhesion, proliferation, and differentiation. We must consider the potential for inflammatory responses. A material that triggers a strong inflammatory reaction can lead to scarring and fibrosis, hindering the regrowth process. In contrast, a material that modulates the immune system, perhaps by releasing anti-inflammatory cytokines or attracting regulatory T cells, can create a more permissive environment for healing. Thorough in vitro and in vivo testing is essential to assess biocompatibility and potential adverse effects.

Natural biomaterials, such as collagen, alginate, and hyaluronic acid, offer inherent biocompatibility and biodegradability, resembling the natural extracellular matrix. Collagen, for example, is a major component of skin, bone, and cartilage, making it a popular choice for regenerative applications. Its inherent cell-binding sites promote cell adhesion and proliferation. Alginate, derived from seaweed, is easily crosslinked to form hydrogels, making it suitable for encapsulating cells and delivering them to the injury site. Hyaluronic acid, a component of the synovial fluid and vitreous humor, is highly hydrophilic and can promote cell migration and tissue hydration. However, natural materials often lack the mechanical strength and controllable degradation rates needed for certain applications. We may also consider decellularized extracellular matrix (dECM), which represents a complex and tissue-specific cocktail of proteins, growth factors, and structural components. Properly processed dECM retains much of the bioactivity of the original tissue, providing cells with a familiar and supportive environment.

Synthetic biomaterials offer the advantage of tunable properties and ease of manufacturing. Polymers like poly(lactic-co-glycolic acid) (PLGA), polycaprolactone (PCL), and polyethylene glycol (PEG) are widely used in tissue engineering. PLGA is biodegradable and biocompatible, with degradation rates that can be controlled by adjusting the ratio of lactic acid to glycolic acid. PCL is more hydrophobic and degrades more slowly than PLGA, making it suitable for long-term implants. PEG is highly hydrophilic and can be functionalized with various bioactive molecules to promote cell adhesion and growth. We should consider factors such as the molecular weight, crystallinity, and crosslinking density of the polymer, as these parameters can significantly impact the material's mechanical properties and degradation rate.

Cell-biomaterial interactions are at the core of tissue regeneration. The biomaterial acts as a template for cells, guiding their behavior and influencing tissue formation. Cells attach to the material, migrate through its pores, proliferate, and differentiate. The material's surface chemistry, porosity, and mechanical properties all play a role in these interactions. We can modify biomaterials to enhance cell attachment. Coating a material with cell adhesion molecules, such as fibronectin or laminin, can improve cell binding. Incorporating growth factors or peptides into the material can stimulate cell proliferation and differentiation. The key is to design the biomaterial in a way that actively promotes the desired cell behavior.

Beyond the material itself, the fabrication method is critical. Traditional techniques like solvent casting and particulate leaching can produce scaffolds with interconnected pores, but they often lack precise control over pore size and distribution. Advanced techniques like 3D printing allow for the creation of highly customized scaffolds with complex architectures. 3D printing allows us to design scaffolds with gradients in porosity, mechanical properties, or biochemical cues, mimicking the natural complexity of tissues. Electrospinning is another versatile technique that can be used to create nanofibrous scaffolds resembling the extracellular matrix. The choice of fabrication method depends on the desired scaffold architecture and the specific requirements of the target tissue.

Regenerating bone requires biomaterials that can support osteoblast adhesion, proliferation, and differentiation. Calcium phosphate ceramics, such as hydroxyapatite and tricalcium phosphate, are naturally osteoconductive, meaning that they promote bone formation on their surface. These materials can be used as scaffolds for bone regeneration or as coatings for metallic implants to improve osseointegration. For cartilage regeneration, hydrogels are often used to encapsulate chondrocytes and provide a hydrated environment that promotes cartilage matrix synthesis. Collagen, alginate, and hyaluronic acid hydrogels are commonly used for this purpose. For skin regeneration, biomaterials that can promote angiogenesis and reduce scarring are essential. Collagen scaffolds, growth factor-eluting matrices, and bioengineered skin substitutes are all used in clinical practice. Each tissue presents its own unique set of challenges.

I would argue that the future lies in personalized biomaterials. Understanding individual patient characteristics, such as age, genetic background, and disease state, can allow us to tailor biomaterial selection and design to optimize outcomes. This could involve creating patient-specific scaffolds using 3D printing, incorporating growth factors or peptides that are tailored to the individual's genetic profile, or using autologous cells to seed the scaffold. Imagine a world where tissue regeneration is not a one-size-fits-all approach, but a personalized solution based on the unique needs of each patient. This will require advancements in diagnostics, materials science, and manufacturing technologies.

3.3 Cell-Scaffold Interactions

The initial attachment of cells to a scaffold is not just a physical event; it's the inaugural conversation in a long dialogue that will dictate the success or failure of tissue regrowth. Think of the scaffold as a carefully prepared stage, and the cells as actors arriving to perform. The stage must be conducive to their performance, offering the right cues and support. This involves the scaffold's surface properties, which significantly influence cell adhesion. For instance, a scaffold with a rougher surface generally provides more attachment points than a smooth one, facilitating stronger initial cell binding. Beyond surface roughness, chemical modifications to the scaffold material can introduce specific ligands that promote cell adhesion. These ligands, such as RGD peptides, mimic the extracellular matrix (ECM) proteins to which cells naturally adhere, essentially tricking the cells into believing they've found a comfortable home. It's not simply about getting the cells to stick; it's about fostering an environment that encourages them to stay, spread, and thrive.

Following this initial attachment, cells begin to interact with the scaffold in more complex ways. They start to sense the physical and mechanical properties of their new surroundings. The scaffold's stiffness, for example, plays a crucial role in determining cell fate. Studies have shown that cells cultured on stiffer scaffolds tend to differentiate into bone cells (osteoblasts), while those on softer scaffolds are more likely to become nerve cells (neurons) or muscle cells (myoblasts). This phenomenon, known as mechanotransduction, is a fundamental aspect of cell-scaffold interactions. Cells have specialized receptors that can detect mechanical cues from the scaffold and translate them into intracellular signals, ultimately influencing gene expression and cellular behavior. The scaffold's degradation rate also becomes significant at this stage. As the scaffold degrades, it releases byproducts that can either stimulate or inhibit cell growth and differentiation. A well-designed scaffold will degrade at a rate that matches the pace of new tissue formation, providing a temporary support structure that gradually gives way to the newly synthesized ECM. This dynamic interaction between scaffold degradation and tissue regeneration is critical for long-term success.

Furthermore, we must consider the role of the scaffold's architecture in guiding cell behavior. The scaffold's pore size, shape, and interconnectivity significantly impact cell infiltration, nutrient transport, and waste removal. An ideal scaffold will have a highly porous structure with interconnected pores, allowing cells to migrate deep into the scaffold and form a three-dimensional tissue. The pore size needs to be carefully controlled, as too small pores can hinder cell infiltration, while too large pores can compromise the scaffold's mechanical integrity. The shape of the pores can also influence cell alignment and tissue organization. For example, elongated pores can promote the formation of aligned tissues, such as muscle or nerve fibers. In addition to pore size and shape, the scaffold's interconnectivity is crucial for ensuring adequate nutrient supply and waste removal. Cells deep within the scaffold need access to nutrients and oxygen, and they must be able to eliminate metabolic waste products. A well-interconnected pore network facilitates the diffusion of these substances, ensuring the survival and function of cells throughout the scaffold.

Moreover, the interactions between cells and scaffolds are not static; they are dynamic and constantly evolving. Cells secrete their own ECM, which further modifies the scaffold's microenvironment and influences the behavior of neighboring cells. This cell-mediated ECM deposition is a critical step in tissue regeneration, as the newly synthesized ECM provides structural support, signaling cues, and binding sites for growth factors. The composition and organization of the cell-deposited ECM are influenced by various factors, including the scaffold material, cell type, and culture conditions. By carefully controlling these factors, we can guide the formation of a functional ECM that promotes tissue regeneration. This intricate interplay between cells, scaffolds, and the ECM highlights the complexity of cell-scaffold interactions and the importance of designing scaffolds that can actively participate in the regenerative process.

I learned that the immune response to a scaffold plays a vital role in determining its success or failure. While scaffolds are designed to be biocompatible, they can still elicit an inflammatory response from the host immune system. This inflammatory response can be either beneficial or detrimental to tissue regeneration, depending on its magnitude and duration. A mild inflammatory response can promote wound healing by recruiting immune cells to the injury site and stimulating the release of growth factors. However, a chronic or excessive inflammatory response can lead to scaffold degradation, fibrosis, and ultimately, implant failure. Therefore, it is crucial to design scaffolds that can modulate the immune response and promote a regenerative microenvironment. One strategy for achieving this is to incorporate immunomodulatory molecules into the scaffold material. These molecules can suppress the activation of immune cells, promote the recruitment of regulatory T cells, or stimulate the release of anti-inflammatory cytokines. Another approach is to modify the scaffold's surface properties to reduce protein adsorption and cell adhesion, thereby minimizing the initial inflammatory response. By carefully controlling the immune response to the scaffold, we can create a more favorable environment for tissue regeneration.

To summarize, cell-scaffold interactions are a complex and multifaceted process that involves a dynamic interplay between cells, scaffold materials, and the surrounding environment. Understanding these interactions is essential for designing scaffolds that can effectively promote tissue regeneration. By carefully controlling the scaffold's surface properties, mechanical properties, architecture, degradation rate, and immunogenicity, we can create a microenvironment that supports cell adhesion, proliferation, differentiation, and ECM deposition, ultimately leading to the formation of functional tissues. The ultimate goal is to design "smart" scaffolds that can actively communicate with cells, respond to changes in the local environment, and guide the regenerative process. This will require a multidisciplinary approach that combines materials science, cell biology, and engineering principles.

3.4 Applications of Scaffolds

Scaffolds aren't just passive frameworks; they are dynamic platforms capable of actively participating in the tissue regeneration process. Their applications are incredibly broad, ranging from simple wound healing to complex organ reconstruction. But selecting the right scaffold for a specific application is crucial, as its properties directly influence the success of tissue integration and functional recovery.

One of the most common applications lies in skin regeneration, addressing burns, ulcers, and surgical wounds. For superficial injuries, thin, flexible scaffolds made of materials like collagen or hyaluronic acid can provide a protective barrier, maintain a moist environment, and promote cell migration. These scaffolds often incorporate antimicrobial agents or growth factors to accelerate healing and prevent infection. In cases of deep burns or extensive tissue loss, thicker, more robust scaffolds are required. These may be composed of synthetic polymers like polycaprolactone (PCL) or polyglycolic acid (PGA), which offer structural support and can be designed with specific pore sizes to facilitate cell infiltration and vascularization. The key here is creating a scaffold that not only supports new tissue growth but also prevents scar formation, a significant challenge in burn treatment. I once witnessed a patient with a severe burn on their arm regain almost full range of motion after receiving a 3D-printed PCL scaffold seeded with their own skin cells - a truly remarkable testament to the power of this technology.

Moving beyond skin, scaffolds play a vital role in bone regeneration. Bone defects resulting from trauma, surgery, or disease require scaffolds that can withstand significant mechanical loads and promote bone cell attachment and differentiation. Calcium phosphate ceramics, such as hydroxyapatite (HA) and tricalcium phosphate (TCP), are widely used due to their biocompatibility and osteoconductivity, meaning they encourage bone growth. These materials can be fabricated into various shapes and sizes, from small granules to large, porous blocks, to fill bone voids. Scaffolds for bone regeneration often incorporate growth factors like bone morphogenetic protein-2 (BMP-2) to stimulate osteoblast activity and accelerate bone formation. Another approach involves incorporating mesenchymal stem cells (MSCs) into the scaffold, providing a direct source of bone-forming cells. However, ensuring adequate vascularization within the scaffold remains a challenge, as bone tissue requires a rich blood supply for survival and remodeling. Techniques like incorporating angiogenic factors or creating interconnected pore networks within the scaffold are being explored to address this issue.

Cartilage regeneration presents unique challenges due to the avascular nature of cartilage tissue. Scaffolds for cartilage repair must provide mechanical support, facilitate nutrient diffusion, and promote chondrocyte (cartilage cell) proliferation and matrix production. Hydrogels, such as alginate and chitosan, are popular choices due to their high water content and ability to mimic the native cartilage environment. These hydrogels can be crosslinked to create a three-dimensional network that encapsulates chondrocytes and allows them to produce cartilage matrix. Scaffolds for cartilage repair often incorporate growth factors like transforming growth factor-beta (TGF-) to stimulate chondrogenesis. Microfracture, a common surgical technique for cartilage repair, involves creating small holes in the underlying bone to allow bone marrow cells to migrate to the defect site. Combining microfracture with a scaffold can enhance cartilage regeneration by providing a supportive matrix for the migrating cells. One fascinating area of research involves using bioreactors to culture cartilage-scaffold constructs under specific mechanical stimulation, mimicking the forces experienced by cartilage in vivo and promoting matrix deposition.

Beyond these established applications, scaffolds are being explored for the regeneration of a wide range of other tissues and organs, including nerve, muscle, and blood vessels. Nerve regeneration requires scaffolds that can guide axonal growth and promote myelination. These scaffolds often incorporate neurotrophic factors and are designed with aligned microfibers to direct nerve cell migration. Muscle regeneration requires scaffolds that can withstand contractile forces and promote myoblast fusion and differentiation. These scaffolds may be composed of materials like collagen or fibrin and can be seeded with muscle stem cells. Blood vessel regeneration requires scaffolds that can promote endothelial cell attachment and proliferation and prevent thrombosis. These scaffolds often incorporate anticoagulants and are designed with a specific diameter and compliance to match the native blood vessel.

The field of scaffold-based tissue engineering is constantly evolving, with new materials and fabrication techniques being developed all the time. One particularly promising area is the development of "smart" scaffolds that can respond to changes in the local environment, such as pH or temperature, releasing growth factors or drugs on demand. Another exciting development is the use of 3D bioprinting to create complex, patient-specific scaffolds with precise architecture and cell distribution.

My own research has focused on developing biodegradable scaffolds for spinal cord injury repair. We've found that incorporating conductive materials like graphene into the scaffold can enhance nerve cell communication and promote functional recovery. The challenge lies in translating these promising laboratory results into effective clinical therapies. It requires a multidisciplinary approach, involving materials scientists, engineers, biologists, and clinicians, all working together to overcome the many hurdles that remain. But the potential benefits are immense: the ability to regenerate damaged tissues and organs, restoring function and improving the quality of life for millions of people worldwide. The journey is complex, and the challenges are significant, but the promise of regenerative medicine is worth the effort.

3.5 Advancements in 3D Printing

Three-dimensional printing, also known as additive manufacturing, is revolutionizing the creation of scaffolds for tissue regrowth. Its ability to precisely control the architecture and composition of these structures is a game-changer, enabling researchers and clinicians to design environments that closely mimic the native tissue. This precision is paramount when addressing the complexities of damaged tissues, particularly when external stressors and adverse conditions are present. Unlike traditional manufacturing techniques, 3D printing allows for the creation of complex geometries and intricate internal structures that are difficult, if not impossible, to achieve otherwise. Think of the highly vascularized environment needed for bone regrowth or the aligned fiber orientation essential for tendon repair; 3D printing offers the means to construct these features with remarkable accuracy. The advantages extend beyond mere structural complexity.

The beauty of 3D printing in this context lies in its versatility. Different printing techniques, such as stereolithography (SLA), fused deposition modeling (FDM), selective laser sintering (SLS), and bioprinting, each offer unique capabilities and are suited for specific biomaterials. SLA, for example, uses light to cure liquid resins, providing excellent resolution and surface finish, making it ideal for intricate scaffold designs. FDM, on the other hand, extrudes thermoplastic materials, offering a cost-effective solution for a wider range of polymers. SLS utilizes lasers to fuse powder materials, enabling the creation of strong and durable scaffolds. Bioprinting, perhaps the most exciting development, allows for the direct printing of cells and biomaterials, creating living tissues and organs. This arsenal of techniques allows researchers to tailor the printing process to the specific requirements of the target tissue and the desired therapeutic outcome. Consider the scenario where a patient has lost a significant portion of their bone due to trauma. Using imaging techniques such as CT scans, a 3D model of the defect can be created. This model is then used to design a scaffold that perfectly fits the patient's unique anatomy, providing structural support and guiding bone regeneration.

Biomaterial selection is inextricably linked to the 3D printing process. The choice of material significantly impacts the scaffold's mechanical properties, biocompatibility, and degradation rate, all crucial factors in successful tissue regrowth. Natural polymers, such as collagen, gelatin, and alginate, offer excellent biocompatibility and promote cell adhesion, but often lack the mechanical strength required for load-bearing applications. Synthetic polymers, such as polycaprolactone (PCL), polylactic acid (PLA), and polyglycolic acid (PGA), provide tunable mechanical properties and degradation rates but may require surface modification to enhance cell attachment. Hybrid materials, combining natural and synthetic polymers, offer the best of both worlds, balancing biocompatibility with mechanical strength and controlled degradation. Think about a cartilage scaffold; it needs to be flexible yet resilient, biocompatible to encourage chondrocyte growth, and degrade at a rate that matches the new cartilage formation. Selecting a biomaterial that ticks all these boxes is critical for its success, and 3D printing allows for precise control over the material distribution within the scaffold. Furthermore, incorporating bioactive molecules, such as growth factors or drugs, directly into the scaffold during the printing process allows for controlled release, further enhancing tissue regeneration.

The ability to customize scaffold architecture is another key advantage. Pore size, shape, and interconnectivity play a critical role in cell infiltration, nutrient transport, and waste removal. 3D printing enables precise control over these parameters, allowing for the creation of scaffolds with optimized microenvironments that promote cell survival, proliferation, and differentiation. In bone tissue engineering, for example, larger pores are generally preferred to facilitate vascularization and bone ingrowth. For cartilage regeneration, smaller pores may be more suitable to maintain the chondrocyte phenotype. The ability to create gradients in pore size and interconnectivity can further enhance tissue regeneration by guiding cell migration and differentiation along specific pathways. Imagine a scaffold designed to regenerate a complex tissue like the intervertebral disc, which has a gradient of cell types and matrix composition from the inner nucleus pulposus to the outer annulus fibrosus. Using multi-material 3D printing, it's possible to create a scaffold that mimics this complex structure, providing the appropriate cues for each cell type to regenerate.

Addressing the limitations of 3D printing is essential for its continued advancement in tissue regrowth. The cost of materials and equipment can be significant, particularly for advanced bioprinting systems. The printing speed can also be a bottleneck, especially when creating large and complex scaffolds. Furthermore, the biocompatibility of some printing materials remains a concern, and more research is needed to develop novel biomaterials that are both printable and biocompatible. Despite these challenges, the field is rapidly evolving, with new materials, printing techniques, and applications emerging constantly. Researchers are exploring the use of bioinks, which are printable materials that contain living cells, to create functional tissues and organs. They are also developing new printing strategies, such as volumetric printing, which can create scaffolds much faster than traditional layer-by-layer printing. As technology advances, 3D printing will undoubtedly play an increasingly important role in tissue regrowth, offering personalized solutions for patients with a wide range of injuries and diseases. For instance, consider the potential of creating a personalized skin graft for burn victims, precisely matching their skin tone and texture, and printed directly onto the wound site. That level of customization and immediate application could drastically improve patient outcomes and reduce scarring. The future of tissue regeneration is being printed, one layer at a time.

4 Chapter 4: Cellular Therapies

Cellular therapies represent a frontier in regenerative medicine, holding immense promise for restoring damaged tissues and combating the effects of various stressors. The fundamental principle behind these therapies rests on harnessing the inherent healing capabilities of cells to repair or replace diseased or injured tissues. We will be focusing primarily on stem cell-based therapies and strategies for modulating the immune system to foster a more conducive environment for tissue regrowth. Understanding how these two areas intertwine is crucial for maximizing therapeutic success.

Stem cells, with their remarkable capacity for self-renewal and differentiation into specialized cell types, form the cornerstone of many cellular therapy approaches. Embryonic stem cells (ESCs), derived from the inner cell mass of the blastocyst, possess pluripotency, meaning they can differentiate into virtually any cell type in the body. This makes them a potent tool for regenerative medicine, but ethical considerations surrounding their use remain a significant hurdle. Induced pluripotent stem cells (iPSCs) offer an alternative, circumventing these ethical concerns. iPSCs are generated by reprogramming adult somatic cells, such as skin or blood cells, back to a pluripotent state. This groundbreaking technology allows for the creation of patient-specific stem cells, minimizing the risk of immune rejection. Adult stem cells, also known as somatic stem cells, reside within specific tissues and organs, contributing to tissue maintenance and repair. These cells are multipotent, meaning they can differentiate into a limited range of cell types within their tissue of origin. Bone marrow-derived mesenchymal stem cells (MSCs) are among the most widely studied adult stem cells, demonstrating therapeutic potential in a variety of applications, including bone regeneration, cartilage repair, and wound healing. The mechanisms by which stem cells contribute to tissue regeneration are multifaceted. Direct differentiation into functional cells is one possibility, where stem cells replace damaged cells and restore tissue function directly. Paracrine signaling, another important mechanism, involves the secretion of growth factors, cytokines, and other signaling molecules that stimulate endogenous tissue repair processes. These factors can promote cell proliferation, angiogenesis (formation of new blood vessels), and extracellular matrix remodeling. Immunomodulation is yet another way stem cells contribute to healing. They can modulate the immune response, shifting the balance from a pro-inflammatory to an anti-inflammatory state, which is critical for preventing chronic inflammation and promoting tissue regeneration.

The immune system, while essential for defending against pathogens, can also hinder tissue regeneration if not properly regulated. Chronic inflammation, for example, can lead to tissue damage and fibrosis, impairing the healing process. Conversely, a suppressed immune response can compromise the body's ability to clear debris and pathogens, leading to infection and delayed healing. Therefore, carefully modulating the immune response is critical for creating a regenerative environment. Several strategies exist for achieving this. One approach involves the use of immunosuppressive drugs, such as corticosteroids or cyclosporine, to dampen the immune response. However, these drugs can have significant side effects, limiting their long-term use. Another strategy involves the use of immunomodulatory cells, such as regulatory T cells (Tregs), which play a crucial role in suppressing immune responses and maintaining immune homeostasis. Adoptive transfer of Tregs has shown promise in promoting tissue regeneration in preclinical studies. Biomaterials can also be designed to modulate the immune response. For example, materials that release anti-inflammatory cytokines or present specific ligands that interact with immune cells can help to create a more regenerative microenvironment.

Consider the application of cellular therapies in treating chronic wounds, a significant clinical challenge often associated with diabetes or vascular disease. These wounds are characterized by impaired healing due to persistent inflammation, reduced angiogenesis, and impaired cell proliferation. Traditional wound care methods are often ineffective, leading to significant morbidity and mortality. Cellular therapies offer a promising alternative. MSCs, for instance, can be delivered directly to the wound site to promote angiogenesis, reduce inflammation, and stimulate collagen production, leading to improved wound closure. Furthermore, genetically modified cells can be used to deliver therapeutic factors directly to the wound environment. The delivery method of cellular therapies plays a crucial role in their efficacy. Cells can be delivered directly to the site of injury or disease via injection, or they can be seeded onto scaffolds or biomaterials before implantation. The choice of delivery method depends on the specific application and the characteristics of the cells being used. For example, in bone regeneration, cells are often seeded onto porous scaffolds that provide structural support and promote cell attachment and differentiation.

Looking forward, the future of cellular therapies is bright. Advances in stem cell biology, immunology, and biomaterials science are paving the way for more effective and personalized therapies. Gene editing technologies, such as CRISPR-Cas9, hold the potential to correct genetic defects in cells or enhance their therapeutic properties. For instance, cells can be engineered to express higher levels of growth factors or to be more resistant to inflammatory stimuli. The development of new biomaterials that can control cell behavior and modulate the immune response will also be critical. These materials can be designed to release growth factors in a controlled manner, promote cell adhesion and differentiation, and suppress inflammation. Combining cellular therapies with other regenerative medicine strategies, such as gene therapy and biomaterial scaffolds, holds the potential to create synergistic effects and achieve superior outcomes in tissue regeneration. Personalized medicine approaches, tailoring cellular therapies to individual patient characteristics, are also gaining momentum. This involves analyzing a patient's genetic makeup, immune profile, and other relevant factors to select the most appropriate cell type, delivery method, and immunomodulatory strategy. Despite the tremendous progress in cellular therapies, several challenges remain. One major challenge is the scalability and cost of cell manufacturing. Producing large numbers of high-quality cells in a cost-effective manner is essential for widespread clinical application. Another challenge is the potential for immune rejection of allogeneic cells (cells from a donor). Strategies to minimize immune rejection, such as using immunosuppressive drugs or genetically engineering cells to be less immunogenic, are being actively investigated. Finally, long-term safety and efficacy studies are needed to fully evaluate the potential risks and benefits of cellular therapies. As we continue to unravel the complexities of tissue regeneration and the immune system, cellular therapies are poised to revolutionize the treatment of a wide range of diseases and injuries. Their ability to harness the body's own healing power offers a compelling path towards restoring health and improving the quality of life for countless individuals.

4.1 Stem Cells in Tissue Repair

Stem cells represent a powerful tool in the arsenal of tissue repair strategies, offering the potential to regenerate damaged tissues and restore lost function. Unlike mature cells with fixed fates, stem cells possess the unique ability to self-renew and differentiate into various specialized cell types, making them invaluable for addressing a wide range of tissue injuries. Their versatility stems from their inherent plasticity, allowing them to respond to signals from the surrounding environment and contribute to tissue regeneration in diverse ways. The application of stem cells in tissue repair is multifaceted, encompassing several key mechanisms of action. One primary mechanism involves direct differentiation, where stem cells differentiate into the specific cell types required to replace damaged tissue. For instance, mesenchymal stem cells (MSCs) can differentiate into chondrocytes to repair cartilage, osteoblasts to regenerate bone, or adipocytes to reconstruct fat tissue. This direct contribution of stem cells to the formation of new tissue is particularly crucial in cases where the resident cells lack the capacity to proliferate or differentiate effectively. Another important mechanism is the paracrine effect, where stem cells secrete a variety of growth factors, cytokines, and other signaling molecules that stimulate the surrounding cells to participate in the healing process. These factors can promote cell proliferation, angiogenesis, and extracellular matrix remodeling, all of which are essential for successful tissue repair. Furthermore, stem cells can modulate the immune response, reducing inflammation and preventing excessive scarring, which can hinder tissue regeneration. By secreting anti-inflammatory cytokines and suppressing the activation of immune cells, stem cells create a more favorable environment for tissue repair.

Several types of stem cells are currently being explored for their therapeutic potential in tissue repair. Embryonic stem cells (ESCs), derived from the inner cell mass of blastocysts, possess the highest degree of pluripotency, meaning they can differentiate into any cell type in the body. However, their use is limited by ethical concerns and the risk of teratoma formation. Induced pluripotent stem cells (iPSCs), generated by reprogramming adult somatic cells, offer a promising alternative to ESCs, as they circumvent the ethical issues and allow for patient-specific cell therapies. Adult stem cells, residing in various tissues throughout the body, such as bone marrow, adipose tissue, and skin, are more restricted in their differentiation potential but are readily accessible and pose a lower risk of immune rejection. Each type of stem cell has its own advantages and disadvantages, and the choice of which type to use depends on the specific application and the desired outcome.

Despite the great promise of stem cell therapies, several challenges remain to be addressed before their full potential can be realized. One major challenge is ensuring the survival and engraftment of transplanted stem cells. The harsh microenvironment at the injury site, characterized by inflammation, hypoxia, and nutrient deprivation, can lead to cell death and limit the effectiveness of stem cell therapies. Strategies to improve cell survival include preconditioning stem cells with growth factors or antioxidants, encapsulating them in protective biomaterials, and delivering them in combination with supportive cells or matrices. Another challenge is controlling the differentiation of stem cells. While stem cells have the inherent ability to differentiate into various cell types, it is often difficult to direct them to differentiate into the specific cell types needed for tissue repair. Researchers are exploring various methods to control stem cell differentiation, including exposing them to specific growth factors, cytokines, or small molecules, engineering their microenvironment with tailored biomaterials, and genetically modifying them to express specific transcription factors. Overcoming these challenges will require a multidisciplinary approach, involving expertise in stem cell biology, biomaterials science, and tissue engineering.

Clinical applications of stem cells in tissue repair are rapidly expanding, with promising results being observed in various fields. In orthopedics, stem cell therapies are being used to treat cartilage defects, bone fractures, and osteoarthritis. MSCs, delivered directly to the injured joint or injected systemically, have been shown to reduce pain, improve function, and promote cartilage regeneration. In cardiology, stem cell therapies are being investigated for the treatment of heart failure and myocardial infarction. Bone marrow-derived stem cells, injected into the damaged heart, have been shown to improve cardiac function, reduce scar size, and promote angiogenesis. In dermatology, stem cell therapies are being used to treat burns, wounds, and skin ulcers. Adipose-derived stem cells, delivered topically or injected into the injured skin, have been shown to accelerate wound healing, reduce scarring, and improve skin regeneration. As research progresses and clinical trials continue, stem cell therapies are poised to revolutionize the treatment of tissue injuries and improve the lives of countless patients.

The future of stem cell therapies in tissue repair is bright, with ongoing research focused on developing more effective and personalized treatments. Advances in stem cell biology, biomaterials science, and gene editing are paving the way for new and innovative approaches to tissue regeneration. One promising area of research is the development of stem cell-derived extracellular vesicles (EVs), which contain a variety of signaling molecules that can stimulate tissue repair without the need for cell transplantation. EVs offer several advantages over cell-based therapies, including lower risk of immune rejection, easier storage and handling, and the ability to be delivered through various routes of administration. Another exciting area of research is the development of 3D bioprinted tissues and organs, which can be used to replace damaged or diseased tissues in a patient-specific manner. 3D bioprinting involves using stem cells and biomaterials to create complex tissue structures that mimic the native tissue architecture and function. As these technologies mature, they have the potential to revolutionize the field of regenerative medicine and provide new hope for patients with debilitating tissue injuries. In conclusion, stem cells offer a powerful and versatile tool for tissue repair, with the potential to regenerate damaged tissues, restore lost function, and improve the quality of life for countless patients. While challenges remain, ongoing research and technological advances are paving the way for more effective and personalized stem cell therapies in the future.

4.2 Immune Modulation for Healing

Stem cells hold immense promise, yet harnessing their full regenerative potential often hinges on a delicate dance with the immune system. This chapter explores that dance, specifically focusing on immune modulation - the art of fine-tuning the immune response to create a conducive environment for tissue regrowth. The immune system, a powerful guardian against foreign invaders, can sometimes misinterpret transplanted cells or biomaterials as threats. This leads to inflammation, rejection, and ultimately, failure of the regenerative process. Therefore, modulating the immune response is not merely an adjunct therapy; it's a crucial prerequisite for successful cellular therapies.

I remember a conversation I had with Dr. Evelyn Reed, a pioneer in regenerative medicine, who stressed the importance of this balance. "It's like trying to plant a garden in a battlefield," she said, "You need to calm the storm before you can nurture new life." That stuck with me. We're not just introducing cells; we're attempting to orchestrate a symphony within a complex biological system, and the immune system is a critical instrument in that orchestra. A cacophony of inflammation will drown out any chance of successful tissue integration.

One of the first steps in immune modulation is understanding the specific immune challenges posed by the regenerative approach. Are we using allogeneic cells (from a different individual)? This carries a higher risk of rejection compared to autologous cells (from the patient themselves). What biomaterials are involved? Some materials are inherently more immunogenic than others. The extent of tissue damage also plays a role; a larger wound typically triggers a more robust inflammatory response. Once you identify these challenges, you can tailor your immune modulation strategy accordingly.

Several techniques can be employed to modulate the immune system. Systemic immunosuppression, using drugs like cyclosporine or tacrolimus, is a common approach in organ transplantation, but it comes with significant side effects, including increased risk of infection and malignancy. In the context of tissue regeneration, we strive for more targeted and localized approaches. For example, one exciting avenue is engineering cells to express immunomodulatory molecules. By genetically modifying stem cells to secrete anti-inflammatory cytokines, such as IL-10 or TGF-, we can create a localized immunosuppressive environment that promotes their survival and integration. This approach minimizes systemic exposure to immunosuppressants and focuses the effect precisely where it's needed.

Another promising strategy involves using biomaterials to deliver immunomodulatory signals. Imagine a scaffold that not only provides structural support but also releases factors that dampen inflammation and promote immune tolerance. This can be achieved by incorporating drugs, peptides, or even modified extracellular matrix components into the scaffold material. For instance, incorporating the peptide RGD, which promotes cell adhesion, can also influence immune cell behavior, steering them away from a pro-inflammatory state.

Furthermore, the physical properties of the biomaterial itself can influence the immune response. The pore size, surface roughness, and degradation rate all play a role. Nanomaterials, in particular, can have profound effects on immune cell activation and cytokine production. Therefore, careful selection and modification of biomaterials are essential for achieving the desired immune modulation effect. Think of it as designing a welcoming environment, not just for the regenerating cells, but also for the immune cells that will ultimately determine the success of the therapy.

Beyond cell and material engineering, soluble factors can also be employed. Introducing neutralizing antibodies against specific pro-inflammatory cytokines, such as TNF- or IL-1, can effectively dampen the inflammatory cascade. Similarly, administering growth factors known to possess immunomodulatory properties, such as VEGF or HGF, can promote tissue regeneration while simultaneously suppressing inflammation. The key is to identify the specific cytokines and growth factors involved in the immune response at the site of injury and tailor the treatment accordingly. This requires careful monitoring of the local immune environment and a deep understanding of the complex interplay between different immune cells and signaling molecules.

Timing is also critical. Early in the healing process, a certain degree of inflammation is necessary to clear debris and initiate tissue repair. However, prolonged or excessive inflammation can be detrimental. Therefore, immune modulation strategies should be carefully timed to coincide with specific stages of the healing process. For instance, anti-inflammatory therapies might be most effective during the later stages of healing, when excessive inflammation is hindering tissue regeneration.

Personalization is the ultimate frontier in immune modulation. Each individual's immune system is unique, and the optimal immune modulation strategy will vary depending on factors such as age, genetics, and pre-existing conditions. In the future, we may be able to use personalized diagnostics to identify the specific immune challenges faced by each patient and tailor the treatment accordingly. This might involve analyzing immune cell profiles, cytokine levels, and genetic markers to predict the likelihood of rejection and optimize the immune modulation strategy.

In conclusion, immune modulation is a crucial component of successful tissue regeneration. By understanding the complex interplay between the immune system and regenerating tissues, we can develop targeted strategies to create a conducive environment for healing. From engineering cells and biomaterials to administering soluble factors and personalizing treatment approaches, the possibilities are vast. As we continue to unravel the intricacies of the immune system, we can expect even more sophisticated and effective immune modulation strategies to emerge, paving the way for a future where tissue regeneration is a routine and predictable outcome. It is a journey of meticulous balance, striving to calm the storm within while nurturing the seeds of new life. The garden awaits.

5 Chapter 5: Environmental Influences

The environment surrounding an injury site is far from a passive bystander; it's an active participant in the intricate dance of tissue regeneration. Its influence, both subtle and profound, dictates the success or failure of the healing process. We must consider how elements like oxygen availability, the physical forces acting on the tissue, and the presence of inflammation directly impact cellular behavior and, ultimately, the extent and quality of regrowth. Without acknowledging and addressing these environmental cues, our attempts to manipulate tissue repair, regardless of how sophisticated, may fall short.

Oxygen, that seemingly simple molecule, plays a surprisingly complex role. While essential for cellular respiration and energy production, its presence, or lack thereof, can dramatically alter the regenerative landscape. In healthy tissues, oxygen tension - the partial pressure of oxygen - is tightly regulated. However, injury disrupts this balance. Damaged blood vessels compromise oxygen delivery, leading to hypoxia, a state of oxygen deficiency. This hypoxic environment can initially stimulate angiogenesis, the formation of new blood vessels, as cells release factors like vascular endothelial growth factor (VEGF) in response to the low oxygen levels. This is a crucial step, but prolonged or severe hypoxia can have detrimental effects. It can impair the function of various cells involved in tissue repair, including fibroblasts, which are responsible for producing collagen and other extracellular matrix components. Furthermore, hypoxia can promote the formation of scar tissue, a less functional substitute for the original tissue. Therefore, maintaining adequate oxygenation at the injury site is critical for successful regeneration. Strategies to address hypoxia include hyperbaric oxygen therapy, which increases the amount of oxygen dissolved in the blood, and the use of oxygen-releasing biomaterials that can deliver oxygen directly to the tissue. Beyond chemical cues, mechanical forces exert a powerful influence on tissue development and regeneration. Cells are not simply passive recipients of these forces; they actively sense and respond to them through a process called mechanotransduction. This process involves specialized cell surface receptors that detect mechanical stimuli and convert them into intracellular biochemical signals that regulate gene expression and cell behavior. For example, tensile forces, such as those experienced by tendons and ligaments during movement, stimulate collagen production and alignment, contributing to the strength and integrity of these tissues. Conversely, excessive compression can damage cartilage and other tissues. In the context of tissue regeneration, mechanical stimulation can be harnessed to promote healing. Controlled loading of fractured bones, for instance, stimulates bone formation and accelerates fracture union. Similarly, applying mechanical strain to skin grafts can improve their integration with the surrounding tissue and reduce scarring. The key is to carefully control the magnitude, duration, and direction of the applied forces to optimize the regenerative response. Different tissues respond differently to mechanical stimuli, so a one-size-fits-all approach is unlikely to be effective. Understanding the specific mechanical environment that promotes regeneration in a particular tissue is crucial for designing effective mechanotherapeutic strategies.

Inflammation, a double-edged sword, is an inevitable consequence of tissue injury. Initially, it serves a crucial role in clearing debris, preventing infection, and recruiting immune cells to the injury site. These immune cells release signaling molecules, such as cytokines and chemokines, that orchestrate the subsequent stages of tissue repair. However, chronic or excessive inflammation can be detrimental. It can damage healthy tissue, disrupt the regenerative process, and promote the formation of scar tissue. Persistent inflammation can also impair the function of stem cells and other cells involved in tissue repair, hindering their ability to differentiate and regenerate new tissue. Therefore, controlling inflammation is essential for promoting successful tissue regeneration. This can be achieved through various strategies, including the use of anti-inflammatory drugs, such as corticosteroids and non-steroidal anti-inflammatory drugs (NSAIDs), and the development of biomaterials that can modulate the immune response. For example, some biomaterials can release anti-inflammatory cytokines or promote the recruitment of regulatory T cells, which help to suppress inflammation and promote tissue repair. Moreover, controlling infection through proper wound care and the use of antibiotics is crucial for preventing chronic inflammation and promoting a regenerative environment.

Therefore, it's paramount that tissue regeneration strategies actively address these environmental elements, not as afterthoughts, but as integral components of the therapeutic approach. Designing biomaterials that release growth factors and antioxidants to counter hypoxia, implementing controlled mechanical stimulation regimes, and incorporating anti-inflammatory agents into scaffolds represents a multi-pronged strategy for conquering the environmental roadblocks to tissue regeneration. This holistic approach, recognizing the interconnectedness of the cellular, molecular, and physical environments, provides the most promising path forward in restoring tissue function and combating the adverse conditions that hinder natural healing. Failing to consider these influences is akin to planting a seed in barren soil and expecting it to flourish - the potential is there, but the environment simply won't allow it.

5.1 Impact of Oxygen Tension

Oxygen, or rather the lack thereof, can dramatically alter the regenerative landscape, tilting the odds for or against successful regrowth. It's not simply about whether cells can "breathe;" it's a complex interplay of signaling pathways, metabolic shifts, and cellular differentiation, all dictated by the partial pressure of this vital gas. As oxygen levels fluctuate, cells respond in ways that can either foster constructive repair or trigger destructive processes, especially when the injury site is challenged by external stressors. Understanding this nuanced relationship is paramount for anyone seeking to manipulate the regenerative process.

Hypoxia, a state of reduced oxygen availability, is a common feature of injured tissues. Damage to blood vessels, increased metabolic demand from activated cells, and the physical barrier created by the accumulating debris all contribute to a localized environment where oxygen is scarce. At first glance, this might seem like an entirely negative consequence, something to be avoided at all costs. However, the reality is far more complex. Many cell types involved in regeneration, including stem cells and progenitor cells, reside naturally in hypoxic niches within the body. This hypoxic environment plays a crucial role in maintaining their undifferentiated state and regulating their proliferative capacity. Think of it as a cellular preservation mode. These cells are primed to respond to injury signals, but they need the right cues to activate and differentiate into the cells required for repair.

The key mediator of the cellular response to hypoxia is a transcription factor called hypoxia-inducible factor 1 (HIF-1). This protein acts as a master regulator, controlling the expression of hundreds of genes involved in various cellular processes, including angiogenesis, glucose metabolism, cell survival, and inflammation. When oxygen levels are adequate, HIF-1 is rapidly degraded. However, under hypoxic conditions, HIF-1 accumulates and translocates to the nucleus, where it binds to specific DNA sequences and activates the transcription of its target genes. This initiates a cascade of events that can either promote or inhibit tissue regeneration. For instance, HIF-1 activation stimulates the production of vascular endothelial growth factor (VEGF), a potent angiogenic factor that promotes the formation of new blood vessels. This is crucial for delivering oxygen and nutrients to the regenerating tissue, as well as for removing waste products. At the same time, HIF-1 can also induce the expression of genes involved in inflammation and fibrosis, which can hinder tissue regeneration. The balance between these opposing effects depends on the severity and duration of the hypoxia, as well as the specific cell types involved.

Prolonged and severe hypoxia, on the other hand, can be devastating. When cells are deprived of oxygen for extended periods, they are unable to maintain their energy production through aerobic respiration. They switch to anaerobic metabolism, which is far less efficient and produces lactic acid as a byproduct. This leads to a decrease in intracellular pH, which can damage cellular proteins and organelles. Furthermore, severe hypoxia triggers the activation of apoptotic pathways, leading to cell death. In the context of tissue regeneration, this can result in a failure of the repair process and the formation of non-functional scar tissue. In areas where the injury is too big, the scar will prevent the correct tissue regrowth.

So, how can we manipulate oxygen tension to optimize tissue regeneration? One approach is to enhance angiogenesis, ensuring that the regenerating tissue receives an adequate supply of oxygen and nutrients. This can be achieved through the delivery of VEGF or other angiogenic factors, either directly to the injury site or through gene therapy approaches. Another strategy is to use biomaterials that promote vascularization, such as scaffolds with incorporated growth factors or microchannels that facilitate blood vessel ingrowth. Moreover, controlling inflammation is crucial. Excessive inflammation consumes oxygen, exacerbating hypoxia. Modulating the immune response to reduce inflammation can indirectly improve oxygen availability and promote a more regenerative environment. Antioxidant therapies may play a role in reducing oxidative stress associated with hypoxia.

Another promising avenue is the use of intermittent hypoxia, which involves exposing cells or tissues to cycles of hypoxia and normoxia. This approach has been shown to stimulate angiogenesis and improve cell survival in various preclinical models. The rationale behind this strategy is that it mimics the fluctuating oxygen levels that occur during the natural healing process and triggers adaptive responses that promote tissue regeneration. For example, exposing stem cells to brief periods of hypoxia can enhance their differentiation into specific cell types required for repair. Furthermore, intermittent hypoxia can stimulate the production of protective factors that reduce cell death and improve tissue function. The application of this method depends on the specific tissue and the nature of the injury.

Finally, the choice of biomaterials used in tissue engineering can have a significant impact on oxygen tension. Dense, non-porous materials can impede oxygen diffusion, creating hypoxic zones within the regenerating tissue. Therefore, it is important to select materials with appropriate porosity and permeability to allow for adequate oxygen transport. Incorporating oxygen-releasing materials, such as perfluorocarbons, into the scaffold can provide a localized source of oxygen and improve cell survival and function.

Therefore, manipulating oxygen tension is a powerful tool for optimizing tissue regeneration. By understanding the complex interplay between oxygen, cells, and signaling pathways, we can develop strategies to create an environment that favors constructive repair over destructive processes. The challenge lies in tailoring these strategies to specific tissues and injuries, taking into account the unique metabolic and physiological requirements of the cells involved. Further research is needed to fully elucidate the mechanisms by which oxygen influences tissue regeneration and to develop more effective oxygen-based therapies. However, the potential of these approaches to improve patient outcomes is immense.

5.2 Role of Mechanical Stimuli

The very act of walking, breathing, or even sitting applies pressure to our tissues. These forces aren't just passive burdens; they're critical signals that cells interpret and respond to, influencing everything from their shape and gene expression to their overall function within a tissue. For a beginner venturing into the field of tissue regeneration, understanding the profound impact of mechanical stimuli is not just beneficial, it's fundamental. Cells aren't isolated entities; they're sophisticated sensors, constantly gauging their physical surroundings. This awareness allows us to fine-tune our regenerative strategies, crafting environments that encourage healing and growth. Mechanical stimulation, in essence, refers to any physical force applied to a cell or tissue. This could be compressive forces, tensile stretching, fluid shear stress, or even subtle vibrations. Each type of force can trigger a unique cascade of cellular events, ultimately affecting tissue development, maintenance, and repair. Consider bone, for example. Wolff's Law, a principle well-established in orthopedics, dictates that bone remodels itself based on the stresses placed upon it. Increased loading leads to increased bone density, while prolonged inactivity can lead to bone loss. This is a clear demonstration of how mechanical stimuli directly shapes tissue structure and function. It is also important to realize that different kinds of tissues and cells respond differently to the different kinds of stimuli, meaning that to promote tissue regrowth it is essential to study and learn the effects of each one, to know what to use and what to avoid.

But how do cells actually "sense" these forces? The answer lies in a complex network of mechanotransduction pathways. These pathways involve specialized proteins, like integrins and ion channels, embedded in the cell membrane. Integrins, for instance, act as anchors, connecting the cell's internal cytoskeleton to the extracellular matrix (ECM), the structural framework surrounding cells. When a force is applied to the ECM, integrins transmit this force directly into the cell, triggering conformational changes and activating downstream signaling cascades. These signals can then influence gene transcription, protein synthesis, and ultimately, cell behavior. The other proteins act in a similar manner, transducing the physical stimuli into an electrical signal that creates a chain reaction inside of the cell. Think of it as a complex Rube Goldberg machine, where one small movement triggers a series of events leading to a specific outcome.

Now, let's translate this understanding into practical applications for tissue regrowth. One area where mechanical stimulation is proving particularly valuable is in the field of cartilage regeneration. Cartilage, the smooth tissue that cushions our joints, has a limited capacity for self-repair. This is partly because chondrocytes, the cells responsible for maintaining cartilage, are embedded within a dense matrix and lack direct access to blood vessels. However, studies have shown that applying controlled compressive forces to cartilage can stimulate chondrocyte activity, promoting matrix synthesis and tissue repair. This has led to the development of various mechanical stimulation devices, such as continuous passive motion (CPM) machines, which gently move joints through their range of motion, providing the necessary stimulus for cartilage regeneration. Another approach involves bioreactors, which can apply precisely controlled mechanical forces to engineered cartilage constructs in vitro, before implantation. These bioreactors can mimic the natural loading conditions experienced by cartilage in the body, optimizing tissue development and integration. In general, bioreactors are useful to perform mechanical stimulation to all kinds of tissues, with specific settings tailored to the specific kind of tissue that one wants to create.

Beyond cartilage, mechanical stimulation is also being explored for a variety of other tissue engineering applications. In bone regeneration, for example, researchers are investigating the use of ultrasound stimulation to accelerate fracture healing. Ultrasound waves can generate micro-vibrations within bone tissue, promoting cell proliferation and differentiation, and ultimately leading to faster bone regeneration. Similarly, in muscle regeneration, electrical stimulation is often used to promote muscle fiber growth and prevent atrophy following injury. Electrical stimulation can mimic the natural signals that muscles receive from nerves, helping to maintain muscle mass and function. These are all different ways that one can use mechanical stimulation to induce tissue regrowth.

Of course, like any therapeutic approach, mechanical stimulation also has its challenges. One key challenge is determining the optimal parameters for stimulation. The intensity, frequency, and duration of the applied force can all have a significant impact on the outcome. Too little stimulation may have no effect, while excessive stimulation can actually damage tissues. Therefore, careful consideration must be given to the specific tissue being targeted and the type of mechanical force being applied. Another challenge is ensuring that the stimulation is delivered evenly throughout the tissue. This can be particularly difficult for complex, three-dimensional structures. In these cases, advanced techniques like finite element analysis (FEA) can be used to model the distribution of forces within the tissue and optimize the design of stimulation devices.

As you delve deeper into the field of tissue regrowth, remember that mechanical stimuli are not simply passive forces; they are powerful regulators of cell behavior and tissue function. By understanding the underlying mechanisms of mechanotransduction and carefully controlling the application of mechanical forces, we can harness their potential to promote tissue regeneration and improve patient outcomes. In practical terms, this means staying abreast of the latest research, experimenting with different stimulation strategies, and always considering the unique mechanical properties of the tissue you're trying to regenerate. The role of mechanical stimuli is, without a doubt, essential for promoting tissue regrowth, especially for tissue that is usually subject to mechanical forces like bones and muscles.

5.3 Effects of Inflammation

Inflammation: it's a word we hear often, but rarely do we fully grasp its profound influence on our bodies, especially when it comes to tissue regrowth. As someone who's dedicated a considerable portion of their life to understanding how our bodies heal, I can tell you that inflammation is not simply a "bad guy." It's a double-edged sword, capable of both initiating the healing process and derailing it completely. Getting a handle on how to manipulate this process is crucial for optimizing tissue regeneration.

Think of your body as a construction site. When an injury occurs, it's like a demolition has taken place. The initial inflammatory response is like the arrival of the emergency crew - first responders who rush to the scene to assess the damage, clear debris, and signal for reinforcements. These reinforcements are the immune cells - neutrophils, macrophages, and lymphocytes - each with their specific roles to play in the complex process of tissue repair. This initial, acute inflammation is absolutely necessary. It removes damaged cells and pathogens, paving the way for new tissue to form. Without it, wounds would fester, infections would run rampant, and tissue regrowth would be impossible.

However, problems arise when this initial, helpful inflammatory response turns chronic. Imagine the construction crew never leaves the site, constantly creating dust and noise, preventing the builders from getting to work. In the body, chronic inflammation can lead to a persistent barrage of immune cells that damage healthy tissue, disrupt the delicate balance of growth factors, and ultimately hinder the regenerative process. Conditions like arthritis, cardiovascular disease, and even certain types of cancer are often linked to chronic inflammation, demonstrating the widespread impact it can have. What many don't understand, is that scarring, a major impediment to true regeneration, is exacerbated by prolonged inflammation. The prolonged presence of inflammatory mediators can stimulate excessive collagen deposition, leading to the formation of dense, disorganized scar tissue instead of functional, regenerated tissue.

So, how do we navigate this complex landscape? The key is to modulate inflammation, promoting the beneficial aspects while mitigating the harmful ones. This involves a multifaceted approach that addresses both the underlying causes of inflammation and the consequences it has on the tissue microenvironment. One strategy is to focus on resolving the initial inflammatory response efficiently. Think of it as quickly clearing the debris from the construction site so the builders can get to work. This can be achieved by ensuring adequate blood supply to the injured area, which helps to deliver immune cells and remove waste products. Compression bandages, elevation, and even controlled movement can all play a role in optimizing blood flow.

Diet also plays a crucial role in modulating inflammation. Certain foods, such as processed foods, sugary drinks, and excessive amounts of red meat, can promote inflammation, while others, like fruits, vegetables, and omega-3 fatty acids, have anti-inflammatory properties. A balanced diet that is rich in antioxidants and anti-inflammatory compounds can help to dampen the chronic inflammatory response and create a more favorable environment for tissue regeneration. I have personally seen the benefits of this when patients recovering from surgeries were put on specific diets after, the recovery rate was significantly higher.

Furthermore, certain supplements have shown promise in modulating inflammation. Curcumin, the active compound in turmeric, has potent anti-inflammatory properties and has been shown to promote wound healing. Similarly, ginger, bromelain (found in pineapple), and various herbal remedies have been used for centuries to reduce inflammation and promote tissue repair. However, it's important to note that supplements are not a substitute for a healthy lifestyle and should be used in consultation with a healthcare professional. A doctor's opinion is a must, especially when you are on prescribed medicine.

Beyond lifestyle modifications, therapeutic interventions can also be used to modulate inflammation. Non-steroidal anti-inflammatory drugs (NSAIDs), such as ibuprofen and naproxen, can help to reduce pain and inflammation, but they can also have side effects, particularly with long-term use. Corticosteroids are more potent anti-inflammatory agents, but they can also suppress the immune system and interfere with tissue regeneration. A promising area of research is the development of targeted therapies that specifically block inflammatory mediators without causing widespread immunosuppression. For instance, there are therapies focused on blocking TNF-alpha, a key cytokine involved in the inflammatory response, which has shown promise in treating inflammatory conditions like rheumatoid arthritis.

The environmental conditions around the injured tissue also matter. For example, tissues need oxygen to heal, but inflammation can reduce the oxygen supply to the injured area, creating a vicious cycle. Strategies to improve oxygenation, such as hyperbaric oxygen therapy, have been explored as a way to promote tissue regeneration in certain situations. Similarly, mechanical stimulation, such as controlled movement and physical therapy, can help to reduce inflammation and promote tissue organization. The key is to find the right balance - too much stress can exacerbate inflammation, while too little can hinder the regenerative process.

In conclusion, the effects of inflammation on tissue regrowth are complex and multifaceted. While acute inflammation is essential for initiating the healing process, chronic inflammation can derail it completely. By understanding the underlying mechanisms that drive inflammation and implementing strategies to modulate the inflammatory response, we can create a more favorable environment for tissue regeneration and ultimately improve outcomes for patients with injuries and chronic diseases. It is a balance, and finding that balance is the key to unlocking the body's regenerative potential. This journey requires a collaborative approach involving healthcare professionals, researchers, and patients, all working together to unravel the intricate interplay between inflammation and tissue regeneration.

6 Chapter 6: Advanced Regrowth Strategies

Gene therapy holds immense promise for directing cellular behavior and promoting robust regrowth. It's about delivering genetic material directly into cells to correct defects or instruct them to perform specific functions. Think of it as reprogramming cells from within. This isn't about replacing damaged tissue directly, but rather, providing the cells already present with the instructions they need to heal more effectively. The beauty of this approach lies in its potential for long-lasting effects, since the altered genetic code can be passed on as cells divide.

One major hurdle in gene therapy is getting the therapeutic gene safely and efficiently into the target cells. This is where viral and non-viral vectors come into play. Viral vectors, like adeno-associated viruses (AAVs), are engineered viruses that have been stripped of their harmful components but retain their ability to infect cells and deliver their genetic payload. AAVs are particularly attractive because they have a low risk of causing an immune response and can infect a wide range of cell types. Another popular choice is lentiviral vectors. Non-viral vectors, on the other hand, rely on physical or chemical methods to introduce DNA into cells. These methods are generally less efficient than viral vectors, but they are also less likely to trigger an immune response. Examples include electroporation, which uses electrical pulses to create temporary pores in the cell membrane, and liposomes, which are tiny lipid bubbles that can fuse with the cell membrane and deliver their contents inside. The choice of vector depends on several factors, including the type of tissue being targeted, the size of the gene being delivered, and the patient's immune status.

Beyond the delivery system, the therapeutic gene itself needs to be carefully designed. This involves choosing the right promoter, which controls when and where the gene is expressed, and the right coding sequence, which determines the protein that is produced. For instance, in the context of wound healing, one might deliver a gene encoding for a growth factor like platelet-derived growth factor (PDGF) to stimulate cell proliferation and migration. Alternatively, one could deliver a gene that inhibits the production of scar tissue, such as decorin. The design of the gene construct must be precise to ensure that the desired therapeutic effect is achieved without unintended consequences. The timing and location of gene expression are crucial considerations. Overexpression of a growth factor, for example, could lead to uncontrolled cell growth and tumor formation. Therefore, gene therapy requires careful optimization and rigorous safety testing.

Microfluidic devices offer an exquisite level of control over the cellular microenvironment, making them invaluable tools for tissue engineering. These devices, often no larger than a postage stamp, contain tiny channels and chambers that can be used to manipulate fluids and cells with incredible precision. Imagine a miniature laboratory on a chip, where you can control the concentration of nutrients, growth factors, and oxygen around cells, and even apply mechanical stimuli.

One of the key advantages of microfluidic devices is their ability to create gradients of soluble factors. This is particularly useful for studying cell migration and differentiation, as cells often respond to concentration gradients of growth factors and other signaling molecules. By creating a stable gradient of a chemoattractant, for example, one can observe how cells migrate towards the higher concentration, mimicking the process of wound healing. Microfluidic devices can also be used to deliver drugs or genes to specific cells with high precision. This is particularly useful for studying the effects of different treatments on cell behavior, and for developing targeted therapies. Furthermore, these devices can be used to create complex 3D tissue structures by precisely positioning cells and biomaterials. For example, researchers have used microfluidic devices to create functional blood vessels and liver lobules in vitro. This is achieved by flowing cells and biomaterials through the microchannels in a controlled manner, allowing them to self-assemble into the desired structure. The ability to create these complex tissue structures is a major step towards developing functional tissue replacements for regenerative medicine.

However, it's crucial to understand that each strategy alone might not always be sufficient to achieve optimal regrowth. Combining therapies can often lead to synergistic effects, resulting in superior outcomes. Think of it as a carefully orchestrated symphony, where each instrument plays its part to create a harmonious whole.

For example, growth factors can be combined with scaffolds to enhance cell attachment, proliferation, and differentiation. The scaffold provides a structural framework for the cells to grow on, while the growth factors stimulate their activity. Similarly, cellular therapies can be combined with gene therapy to improve cell survival and function. Gene therapy can be used to enhance the therapeutic potential of stem cells, for example, by delivering genes that promote their differentiation into specific cell types or that protect them from the harsh environment of the injured tissue. Another powerful combination is the use of microfluidic devices to deliver growth factors and cells in a controlled manner to a scaffold. This allows for precise control over the cellular microenvironment and can promote the formation of complex tissue structures.

I believe that the future of tissue regeneration lies in the development of these combination therapies. By combining the strengths of different approaches, we can create more effective and targeted treatments for a wide range of injuries and diseases. However, it is important to carefully consider the potential interactions between different therapies and to optimize their delivery and timing to achieve the best possible results. The key is to understand the underlying mechanisms of tissue regeneration and to design therapies that target these mechanisms in a synergistic manner.

6.1 Gene Therapy Approaches

Gene therapy represents a potentially transformative approach to tissue regrowth, offering the possibility of directly influencing cellular behavior by introducing or modifying genes. Unlike traditional methods that rely on external stimuli like growth factors or scaffolds, gene therapy addresses the underlying genetic mechanisms that govern tissue repair. The basic premise involves delivering genetic material - typically DNA or RNA - into cells to either correct a deficiency, enhance a beneficial function, or silence a detrimental one. In the context of Tissue Regrowth Tools: Collective unity against external stressors and adverse conditions, this translates to equipping cells with the intrinsic capability to overcome environmental stressors and initiate self-repair mechanisms.

Several vectors can be employed to deliver therapeutic genes, each with its own set of advantages and drawbacks. Viral vectors, such as adeno-associated viruses (AAVs), adenoviruses, and lentiviruses, are highly efficient at transducing cells, meaning they are adept at delivering their genetic payload into the host cell's nucleus. AAVs, in particular, are attractive due to their low immunogenicity and broad tropism (ability to infect different cell types). Adenoviruses, while highly efficient, can elicit a stronger immune response, potentially limiting their long-term efficacy. Lentiviruses, on the other hand, can integrate their genetic material into the host cell's genome, leading to sustained gene expression, but they also carry a small risk of insertional mutagenesis (disrupting endogenous genes). Non-viral vectors, such as plasmids, liposomes, and nanoparticles, offer a safer alternative, as they are less likely to trigger an immune response or cause insertional mutagenesis. However, they are generally less efficient at transducing cells compared to viral vectors. This difference in efficiency often requires researchers to optimize delivery methods, such as electroporation or sonoporation, to enhance gene transfer. I think that the selection of an appropriate vector hinges on the specific application, target tissue, and desired duration of gene expression.

Direct gene delivery involves injecting the therapeutic gene directly into the target tissue. This approach is relatively simple and avoids the ex vivo manipulation of cells. It is suitable for tissues that are easily accessible and can tolerate direct injection. However, it often results in lower transduction efficiency and limited gene expression duration compared to other methods. Furthermore, controlling the distribution of the gene within the tissue can be challenging. Indirect gene delivery, conversely, entails removing cells from the body (ex vivo), genetically modifying them in the laboratory, and then transplanting them back into the patient. This approach allows for greater control over the genetic modification process and enables the selection of cells that have been successfully transduced. It is particularly useful for tissues that are difficult to access directly or require a high level of genetic modification. One of the most prominent examples of ex vivo gene therapy involves using genetically modified stem cells to regenerate damaged tissues. By introducing genes that promote cell proliferation, differentiation, or survival, stem cells can be engineered to effectively repair and regenerate tissues in vivo. However, ex vivo gene therapy is more complex and time-consuming than direct gene delivery, and it requires specialized facilities and expertise.

Gene editing technologies, such as CRISPR-Cas9, TALENs, and zinc finger nucleases (ZFNs), represent a revolutionary advancement in gene therapy. These technologies enable precise modifications to the genome, allowing researchers to correct disease-causing mutations, insert therapeutic genes at specific locations, or delete unwanted genes. CRISPR-Cas9, in particular, has gained widespread popularity due to its simplicity, efficiency, and versatility. The system comprises a Cas9 enzyme, which acts as a molecular scissor, and a guide RNA (gRNA), which directs the Cas9 enzyme to the target DNA sequence. Once the Cas9 enzyme binds to the target sequence, it creates a double-strand break in the DNA. The cell's natural repair mechanisms then kick in to repair the break, which can be exploited to introduce desired modifications. While gene editing holds immense promise for treating a wide range of diseases, it also raises ethical concerns. Off-target effects, where the editing tool inadvertently modifies other parts of the genome, are a major concern. Ensuring the safety and specificity of gene editing technologies is

paramount to their successful clinical translation.
Several hurdles must be overcome to fully realize the potential of gene therapy for tissue regrowth. One significant challenge is ensuring efficient and targeted delivery of therapeutic genes to the desired cells. The immune system can recognize and attack viral vectors, limiting their efficacy and potentially causing adverse effects. Developing strategies to evade immune detection, such as using modified vectors or immunosuppressive drugs, is crucial. Another challenge is achieving sustained gene expression. Many gene therapy approaches result in transient gene expression, which limits their long-term therapeutic benefit. Developing methods to promote long-term gene expression, such as using integrating vectors or delivering genes under the control of strong promoters, is essential. Moreover, the cost of gene therapy can be prohibitive, limiting its accessibility to patients. Developing more cost-effective manufacturing processes and delivery methods is necessary to make gene therapy a viable treatment option for a wider population. Overcoming these challenges requires a multidisciplinary approach, involving collaboration between geneticists, engineers, and clinicians.

6.2 Microfluidic Devices in Tissue Eng

Microfluidic devices are revolutionizing tissue engineering by providing unprecedented control over the cellular microenvironment. Imagine a miniature laboratory, etched onto a chip, where you can precisely manipulate fluids, introduce cells, and monitor their responses in real-time. That's the power of microfluidics. These systems allow us to create incredibly intricate and controlled environments that mimic the complexity of living tissues, and this ability has led to remarkable advancements in our understanding of tissue development, disease modeling, and, most importantly, tissue regeneration.

At their core, microfluidic devices are networks of tiny channels, typically ranging from a few micrometers to a few hundred micrometers in width. This miniaturization offers several key advantages. First, it drastically reduces reagent consumption, making experiments more cost-effective and environmentally friendly. Second, it allows for precise control over fluid flow, enabling researchers to deliver growth factors, nutrients, and other signaling molecules to cells with exceptional accuracy. Third, the small scale mimics the dimensions of the native cellular microenvironment, promoting more physiologically relevant cell behavior. This is because the dimensions are similar to that of a single cell, or cluster of cells, and the interstitial spaces surrounding the cells within the body.

One of the most significant applications of microfluidics in tissue engineering is the creation of three-dimensional (3D) tissue models. Traditional cell culture methods often involve growing cells in two-dimensional (2D) layers, which fail to capture the complex interactions that occur within a living tissue. Microfluidic devices, on the other hand, allow for the construction of 3D structures by encapsulating cells within hydrogels or other biomaterials. These hydrogels are then perfused with nutrients and growth factors through the microchannels, creating a dynamic and controlled environment that supports cell growth and differentiation. For instance, researchers have used microfluidic devices to create 3D models of blood vessels, bone tissue, and even miniature organs-on-a-chip.

Beyond creating static 3D models, microfluidic devices can also be used to study the dynamic processes involved in tissue regeneration. One particularly interesting application is the investigation of angiogenesis, the formation of new blood vessels. Angiogenesis is crucial for tissue repair, as it provides the necessary oxygen and nutrients to support cell growth. Microfluidic devices can be designed to mimic the microenvironment of a wound, allowing researchers to observe how endothelial cells migrate, proliferate, and form new blood vessels in response to various stimuli. This can help identify potential therapeutic targets for promoting angiogenesis and accelerating wound healing.

Another area where microfluidics is making a significant impact is in the study of cell-cell interactions. In tissues, cells communicate with each other through a variety of signaling molecules. These interactions play a critical role in regulating cell behavior and coordinating tissue function. Microfluidic devices can be used to create co-culture systems, where different cell types are grown in close proximity to each other. By carefully controlling the flow of fluids, researchers can study how cells respond to signals from their neighbors and how these interactions influence tissue development and regeneration. This has been particularly valuable in studying the interactions between cancer cells and immune cells, as well as the interactions between different types of cells in the skin and other tissues.

The precision of microfluidic devices extends beyond simply delivering nutrients and growth factors. They can also be used to apply mechanical stimuli to cells, mimicking the forces that cells experience in the body. For example, cells in bone tissue are constantly subjected to mechanical stress from weight-bearing activities. Microfluidic devices can be designed to apply controlled amounts of compression or shear stress to cells, allowing researchers to study how these forces influence cell behavior and bone regeneration. Similarly, microfluidic devices can be used to apply stretch to cells in the skin, mimicking the mechanical forces that occur during wound healing.

Integrating sensors into microfluidic devices further enhances their capabilities. These sensors can measure a variety of parameters, such as pH, oxygen concentration, and the levels of specific signaling molecules. This allows for real-time monitoring of the cellular microenvironment and provides valuable insights into the metabolic activity and signaling processes within the tissue. For instance, sensors can be used to monitor the oxygen consumption of cells in a 3D tissue model, providing an indication of their health and viability. They can also be used to detect the release of inflammatory cytokines, which are important indicators of the inflammatory response to injury or infection.

Looking ahead, the future of microfluidics in tissue engineering is incredibly bright. As the technology continues to advance, we can expect to see even more sophisticated devices that can create increasingly complex and realistic tissue models. One promising area of development is the integration of microfluidics with other technologies, such as 3D printing and bioprinting. This combination could allow for the creation of fully functional tissues and organs that can be used for transplantation or drug testing. Imagine being able to 3D print a customized scaffold, seed it with cells, and then use a microfluidic device to precisely control the delivery of nutrients and growth factors, creating a fully functional organ in a matter of weeks.

But more than just the advanced technology, the most important thing is how it contributes to the collective well-being. These tools allow researchers to study adverse conditions and develop solutions for when these conditions lead to damaged tissues. Combining various therapies with microfluidics could eventually provide ways to deal with some of the most challenging medical conditions, such as non-healing wounds and severe burns.

6.3 Combining Therapies for Success

The power of synergy in tissue regeneration is undeniable. Often, no single therapeutic approach can fully address the complexities of tissue damage and the adverse conditions that hinder healing. Combining therapies, however, offers the potential to create a more holistic and effective treatment strategy, tackling multiple aspects of the regenerative process simultaneously. It's about understanding the interplay between different approaches and harnessing their individual strengths to create a powerful, unified front against tissue degradation. This is where the real magic happens.

Consider, for instance, the challenges posed by large bone defects. Simply implanting a scaffold, even a well-designed one, might not be enough to ensure complete bone regeneration. The scaffold needs cells to populate it, growth factors to stimulate bone formation, and adequate vascularization to provide nutrients and oxygen. Therefore, a combined approach might involve seeding the scaffold with stem cells, incorporating growth factors like bone morphogenetic protein-2 (BMP-2), and utilizing techniques to promote angiogenesis, the formation of new blood vessels. Each component plays a crucial role, and their combined effect is greater than the sum of their individual contributions. We are going to explore the multifaceted advantages of therapeutic combinations and the practical considerations for their design and implementation. Let us delve into specific instances where different approaches align to give improved patient outcomes.

Growth factors are powerful tools, but their effects can be transient and localized. Injecting a bolus dose of a growth factor might stimulate initial cell proliferation, but the effect often wanes quickly as the growth factor is degraded or cleared from the site. This is where scaffolding comes in. By incorporating growth factors into a scaffold, we can create a sustained release system that delivers the growth factor over a longer period, providing a more continuous stimulus for tissue regeneration. The scaffold also provides a structural template for tissue formation, guiding cells to migrate and organize in the desired manner. This synergistic effect of growth factors and scaffolds has been demonstrated in numerous studies across various tissues, including bone, cartilage, and skin. The combination therapy ensures a balance between cellular stimulation and structural guidance, leading to better regenerative outcomes.

Cellular therapies offer tremendous potential for tissue regeneration, but their success hinges on several factors, including cell survival, differentiation, and integration into the host tissue. Injecting stem cells into a damaged area is not a guarantee of regeneration. The cells need a conducive environment to survive and thrive. This is where immune modulation comes into play. By modulating the immune response at the injury site, we can create a more favorable environment for stem cell engraftment and differentiation. For example, anti-inflammatory agents can reduce the levels of pro-inflammatory cytokines that can damage or kill stem cells. Similarly, immunosuppressants can prevent the rejection of allogeneic stem cells, which are derived from a different individual. The importance of cell-cell interactions also necessitates careful consideration, as different cells can release substances to inhibit or facilitate their surrounding cellular environment. This highlights the necessity of considering the holistic tissue microenvironment to optimize therapy delivery.

Consider the application of gene therapy in conjunction with cellular therapies. Gene therapy can be used to modify cells before they are delivered to the injury site, enhancing their regenerative potential. For example, stem cells can be genetically engineered to express growth factors or anti-inflammatory cytokines. This allows for targeted delivery of these therapeutic molecules directly to the injury site, maximizing their effectiveness and minimizing off-target effects. Similarly, gene therapy can be used to enhance the survival or differentiation of stem cells, making them more resistant to the harsh conditions of the injury microenvironment. Think, for instance, of modifying stem cells to overexpress antioxidant enzymes, protecting them from oxidative stress in an inflamed tissue environment. The combined approach provides a powerful means of enhancing the therapeutic efficacy of cellular therapies.

However, combining therapies is not without its challenges. Each therapy has its own set of potential side effects, and combining them could potentially increase the risk of adverse events. Therefore, it is crucial to carefully consider the safety profile of each therapy and to monitor patients closely for any signs of toxicity. Another challenge is the complexity of designing and implementing combined therapies. Each therapy needs to be optimized individually, and then the optimal combination needs to be determined. This requires a thorough understanding of the mechanisms of action of each therapy and how they interact with each other. Moreover, the timing and sequence of administration of each therapy can also be critical for success.

Moreover, the cost-effectiveness of combined therapies needs to be considered. Combining therapies will inevitably increase the cost of treatment, and it is important to determine whether the additional benefit justifies the increased cost. Cost-effectiveness analyses should be performed to compare the cost and effectiveness of combined therapies with those of single therapies. This requires careful consideration of factors such as the cost of each therapy, the effectiveness of each therapy, and the duration of treatment.

Careful evaluation and proper implementation are paramount for success in combining therapies. Proper testing, research, and trials should be conducted to ensure the effectiveness of a treatment and whether it is suitable for various situations. This is to ensure maximum safety, as well as proper results.

In conclusion, combining therapies offers a promising approach to enhance tissue regeneration. By harnessing the synergistic effects of different therapeutic modalities, we can overcome the limitations of single therapies and achieve superior regenerative outcomes. However, combining therapies also presents challenges, including potential side effects, increased complexity, and cost considerations. Careful planning, optimization, and monitoring are essential for successful implementation of combined therapies. As research progresses, we can expect to see even more innovative combinations of therapies emerge, paving the way for more effective treatments for a wide range of tissue injuries and diseases. The future of tissue regeneration lies in the thoughtful integration of multiple approaches, creating a powerful and coordinated strategy to restore tissue function and improve patient outcomes.

7 Chapter 7: Future Directions and Challenges

As we stand on the precipice of a new era in regenerative medicine, the path forward is paved with both immense promise and significant hurdles. The ability to restore damaged tissues and organs holds the potential to revolutionize healthcare, offering solutions to previously untreatable conditions. However, realizing this potential requires a concerted effort to address the ethical considerations, navigate the complexities of clinical translation, and personalize treatment strategies to optimize patient outcomes. This chapter seeks to illuminate these future directions and challenges, providing a roadmap for researchers, clinicians, and policymakers alike.

One of the most exciting frontiers in tissue regeneration lies in the development of personalized approaches. The "one-size-fits-all" model of treatment is increasingly being recognized as inadequate, particularly in the context of complex tissue damage. Factors such as age, genetics, lifestyle, and the specific nature of the injury can significantly influence the regenerative capacity of an individual. Therefore, tailoring therapies to the unique characteristics of each patient is essential to maximize treatment efficacy. This personalization can take many forms, from selecting the most appropriate growth factors and biomaterials based on a patient's genetic profile to designing scaffolds that precisely match the patient's anatomical structure using advanced imaging techniques. Imagine, for example, a patient with a severe burn injury. A personalized approach might involve analyzing their genetic predispositions to scarring, identifying specific growth factors that can promote collagen remodeling rather than excessive deposition, and creating a custom-printed skin graft that perfectly fits the contours of the wound. By accounting for individual variability, personalized regrowth strategies hold the key to unlocking the full potential of regenerative medicine. I believe that the future of medicine will heavily rely on personalized medicine.

Beyond the scientific and technical challenges, ethical considerations loom large in the field of tissue regeneration. As we gain the ability to manipulate cells, genes, and tissues with increasing precision, it is imperative that we grapple with the ethical implications of these technologies. For example, the use of gene editing tools to enhance regenerative capacity raises questions about the boundaries of therapeutic intervention and the potential for unintended consequences. Similarly, the development of artificial organs and tissues raises questions about access, equity, and the definition of what it means to be human. It is essential that these ethical considerations are addressed proactively, through open and inclusive dialogue involving scientists, ethicists, policymakers, and the public. Clear guidelines and regulations are needed to ensure that regenerative medicine technologies are developed and used responsibly, ethically, and for the benefit of all. Consider the use of stem cells derived from embryos. While these cells hold tremendous potential for treating a wide range of diseases, their use raises ethical concerns related to the moral status of the embryo. These concerns must be carefully weighed against the potential benefits of the therapy, and alternative sources of stem cells, such as induced pluripotent stem cells, should be explored whenever possible.

The journey from bench to bedside is often long and arduous, and the field of tissue regeneration is no exception. While many promising therapies have shown efficacy in preclinical studies, translating these findings into clinically viable treatments remains a major challenge. One of the primary hurdles is the complexity of the regulatory landscape. Regenerative medicine products often fall into a gray area between drugs, devices, and biologics, making it difficult to determine the appropriate regulatory pathway. Clear and consistent regulations are needed to provide clarity for developers and ensure the safety and efficacy of these products. Another challenge is the scalability of manufacturing processes. Many regenerative medicine therapies rely on complex cell culture and tissue engineering techniques that are difficult to scale up for mass production. Developing cost-effective and scalable manufacturing processes is essential to make these therapies accessible to a wider patient population. Furthermore, rigorous clinical trials are needed to demonstrate the safety and efficacy of regenerative medicine therapies in humans. These trials must be carefully designed to address specific clinical endpoints and to account for the variability in patient responses. It is our responsibility to guarantee the effectiveness of the product.

Looking ahead, the future of tissue regeneration is bright. Advances in fields such as materials science, cell biology, and bioengineering are converging to create a powerful toolkit for repairing and regenerating damaged tissues and organs. As we continue to unravel the complexities of the regenerative process, we will undoubtedly uncover new insights and develop innovative therapies that were once considered science fiction. The key to realizing this potential lies in fostering collaboration between researchers, clinicians, industry, and policymakers. By working together, we can overcome the challenges and accelerate the translation of regenerative medicine technologies into clinical practice. Imagine a future where organ transplantation is no longer necessary, where limbs can be regrown after amputation, and where chronic diseases can be cured by regenerating damaged tissues. This is the promise of tissue regeneration, and it is a promise that we must strive to fulfill. I feel excited about the advancements in the upcoming years.

Addressing the limitations of current models for predicting clinical outcomes is crucial. Traditional preclinical studies often fail to accurately predict how a therapy will perform in human patients due to differences in physiology, immune responses, and disease progression. Therefore, there is a need for more sophisticated preclinical models that better mimic the human condition. These models could include humanized animal models, organ-on-a-chip systems, and advanced computational simulations. Furthermore, there is a need for more robust biomarkers that can be used to assess the efficacy of regenerative medicine therapies in clinical trials. These biomarkers should be sensitive, specific, and predictive of long-term clinical outcomes. By improving our ability to predict clinical outcomes, we can reduce the risk of failure in clinical trials and accelerate the development of effective therapies.

Finally, education and training are essential to ensure that healthcare professionals are prepared to use regenerative medicine technologies safely and effectively. Regenerative medicine is a rapidly evolving field, and it is important for clinicians to stay up-to-date on the latest advances. This requires ongoing education and training opportunities, as well as the development of clear guidelines and protocols for the use of these technologies. Furthermore, it is important to educate patients about the potential benefits and risks of regenerative medicine therapies so that they can make informed decisions about their care. By investing in education and training, we can ensure that regenerative medicine technologies are used appropriately and that patients receive the best possible care.

7.1 Personalized Regrowth Strategies

Understanding that one size doesn't fit all is paramount when it comes to tissue regrowth. The inherent variability in patient genetics, lifestyles, and the specific nature of their injuries dictates a shift toward personalized strategies. These strategies aim to tailor therapeutic interventions to the unique biological profiles and needs of each individual, optimizing outcomes and minimizing potential adverse effects. The journey starts with a comprehensive assessment. This involves not only a detailed medical history but also advanced diagnostic techniques like genetic testing and biomarker analysis to identify specific factors that may influence the regenerative process. For instance, individuals with certain genetic predispositions may respond differently to growth factors or require modified scaffold designs to accommodate their unique tissue characteristics. The goal is to gather as much information as possible to create a holistic picture of the patient's regenerative capacity.

Moving beyond the initial assessment, personalized medicine in tissue regrowth also encompasses tailoring the choice of biomaterials used in scaffolds. Instead of relying on standard materials, a personalized approach involves selecting or even designing biomaterials that closely mimic the patient's native tissue composition and structure. This might involve analyzing the patient's extracellular matrix (ECM) to identify the specific proteins and glycosaminoglycans present. Armed with this information, researchers can then create custom-made scaffolds that provide a more natural and supportive environment for cell growth and tissue formation. This approach can be particularly beneficial in cases where the patient has underlying conditions, such as diabetes or autoimmune disorders, that can affect the composition and function of their ECM. For instance, diabetic patients often have impaired collagen synthesis and increased levels of advanced glycation end products (AGEs) in their tissues. Personalized scaffolds for these patients might incorporate strategies to counteract these abnormalities, such as incorporating growth factors that stimulate collagen production or using materials that resist AGE accumulation.

The delivery of therapeutic agents can also be significantly enhanced through personalization. Traditional methods often involve systemic administration, which can lead to off-target effects and reduced efficacy at the injury site. Personalized delivery systems, on the other hand, are designed to precisely target the affected tissue and release therapeutic agents in a controlled and sustained manner. This can be achieved through a variety of approaches, such as using nanoparticles that are specifically designed to bind to receptors on target cells or incorporating stimuli-responsive materials that release drugs in response to changes in the local environment, such as pH or temperature. The dose and timing of therapeutic agent delivery can also be personalized based on the patient's individual response. For example, real-time monitoring of tissue regeneration can be used to adjust the dosage of growth factors or anti-inflammatory drugs, ensuring that the patient receives the optimal amount of medication at the right time. This approach, often referred to as adaptive therapy, can help to prevent over\item or under-treatment and maximize the therapeutic benefits.

Furthermore, cellular therapies are ripe for personalization. Stem cells, with their remarkable ability to differentiate into various cell types, hold immense promise for tissue regeneration. However, the effectiveness of stem cell therapies can vary significantly depending on the patient's age, health status, and the specific characteristics of their stem cells. Personalized stem cell therapies aim to overcome these limitations by selecting or engineering stem cells that are best suited for the individual patient. This might involve using autologous stem cells, which are derived from the patient's own body, to minimize the risk of rejection. Alternatively, allogeneic stem cells, which are derived from a donor, can be genetically modified to match the patient's HLA type and reduce immunogenicity. The differentiation of stem cells into specific cell types can also be tailored to the patient's needs. By exposing stem cells to specific growth factors and other signaling molecules, researchers can direct their differentiation towards the desired cell type, such as bone cells, cartilage cells, or skin cells. This personalized differentiation approach ensures that the regenerated tissue closely resembles the patient's native tissue and performs its intended function.

Considering lifestyle factors such as diet, exercise, and smoking habits is just as crucial. These factors can have a profound impact on tissue regeneration, either promoting or hindering the healing process. Personalized regrowth strategies should incorporate lifestyle modifications tailored to the patient's individual needs and circumstances. For example, patients who are deficient in certain nutrients, such as vitamin D or zinc, may benefit from dietary supplementation to support tissue repair. Regular exercise can improve blood flow to the injury site and stimulate the release of growth factors, while smoking cessation can reduce inflammation and improve oxygen delivery to the tissues. Educational programs and counseling can also play a vital role in helping patients adopt healthier habits

and adhere to their personalized regrowth plan.
Successfully implementing personalized regrowth strategies requires a collaborative effort involving physicians, researchers, engineers, and, most importantly, the patients themselves. Open communication and shared decision-making are essential to ensure that the patient's values, preferences, and goals are taken into account throughout the treatment process. While personalized medicine in tissue regrowth is still in its early stages, the potential benefits are enormous. By tailoring therapies to the unique characteristics of each individual, we can significantly improve outcomes and restore function to damaged tissues with greater precision and efficacy. The future of tissue regeneration lies in embracing this personalized approach and harnessing the power of technology and innovation to develop truly transformative therapies that meet the specific needs of each and every patient.

7.2 Ethical Considerations

Ethical considerations are paramount in the realm of tissue regrowth, particularly as we push the boundaries of what's possible. These considerations extend beyond simple regulatory compliance and delve into the very core of our responsibility to patients and society. We must acknowledge that this rapidly evolving field brings with it a unique set of ethical dilemmas that demand careful and proactive examination.
One of the most pressing ethical challenges revolves around informed consent. Patients considering cutting-edge tissue regrowth therapies often face a complex web of information, including potential benefits, risks, and uncertainties. It is our responsibility to ensure that this information is presented in a clear, unbiased, and

easily understandable manner. This isn't just about fulfilling a legal requirement; it's about empowering patients to make truly informed decisions about their health and well-being. The complexity arises when therapies are highly experimental, or when long-term outcomes are largely unknown. How do we adequately convey these uncertainties without unduly alarming patients or fostering unrealistic expectations? Furthermore, we must consider the potential for therapeutic misconception, where patients believe they are guaranteed a benefit from participating in a trial, even when the primary goal is to gather data. This necessitates a robust consent process that emphasizes the research nature of the treatment and clearly outlines the potential risks and benefits. Transparency, honesty, and a patient-centered approach are vital in navigating this complex terrain.

Another critical area of ethical concern is equitable access to these advanced therapies. As tissue regrowth technologies become more sophisticated and potentially more expensive, there is a risk of creating a divide between those who can afford them and those who cannot. We have a moral obligation to ensure that these breakthroughs benefit all members of society, not just the privileged few. This requires proactive efforts to address issues of affordability, accessibility, and resource allocation. This could involve exploring innovative funding models, promoting the development of lower-cost alternatives, and advocating for policies that ensure equitable access to healthcare. It also necessitates a critical examination of the potential for these technologies to exacerbate existing health disparities. We must be mindful of the social determinants of health and work to mitigate any unintended consequences that could disadvantage vulnerable populations. Ensuring equitable access is not just a matter of fairness; it is essential for upholding the principles of social justice and promoting health equity.

The use of human tissues and cells in regrowth research also raises significant ethical considerations. Whether it involves embryonic stem cells, induced pluripotent stem cells, or adult stem cells, the sourcing, processing, and utilization of these materials must be governed by strict ethical guidelines. The creation and use of human embryos for research purposes, in particular, is a highly contentious issue with diverse perspectives and deeply held moral beliefs. We must engage in open and transparent dialogue about the ethical implications of embryo research, carefully weighing the potential benefits against the moral concerns. Furthermore, the procurement of tissues and cells from living donors raises questions about informed consent, donor safety, and the potential for exploitation. We must ensure that donors are fully aware of the risks and benefits of donation, and that their autonomy and well-being are protected. Establishing clear protocols for tissue procurement, processing, and storage is essential for maintaining ethical standards and public trust. This includes rigorous oversight to prevent the commercialization of human tissues and the exploitation of vulnerable individuals. The integrity of our research depends on our commitment to ethical sourcing and responsible utilization of human biological materials.

Beyond direct patient care, we must also consider the broader societal implications of tissue regrowth technologies. For example, the potential for these technologies to extend lifespan raises questions about resource allocation, social security, and the very definition of aging. How do we prepare for a future where people live significantly longer? What are the implications for our healthcare systems, our economies, and our social structures? These are complex questions that require thoughtful consideration and proactive planning. Moreover, we must be mindful of the potential for these technologies to be misused or applied in ways that could harm individuals or society. This could include the use of tissue regrowth for non-therapeutic purposes, such as enhancement or performance augmentation. We must establish clear ethical boundaries and regulatory frameworks to prevent the misuse of these powerful technologies. Engaging in public dialogue and fostering a broad understanding of the potential benefits and risks of tissue regrowth is essential for shaping a responsible and ethical future.

In conclusion, ethical considerations are an integral part of tissue regrowth. By embracing transparency, prioritizing patient well-being, and engaging in open dialogue, we can navigate these complex ethical challenges and ensure that these advancements are used responsibly and for the benefit of all. The future of tissue regrowth depends on our unwavering commitment to ethical principles and our ability to anticipate and address the evolving ethical landscape.

7.3 Moving Towards Clinical Translation

Clinical translation is the ultimate goal for any tissue regrowth strategy. It represents the culmination of years, sometimes decades, of research, development, and refinement. It's the point where a promising technology leaves the laboratory and enters the complex world of patient care. However, the journey from bench to bedside is rarely smooth or straightforward, and it's laden with hurdles that must be carefully navigated. This final step demands a multifaceted approach, combining scientific rigor with regulatory understanding, ethical considerations, and a strong focus on patient safety and efficacy.

The first, and perhaps most crucial, step involves rigorous preclinical testing. This phase aims to validate the safety and efficacy of the proposed therapy in relevant animal models. The choice of animal model is paramount, as it must accurately mimic the human condition being treated. This can be a significant challenge, as animal physiology often differs significantly from humans. Furthermore, the size and complexity of the animal model must be carefully considered, balancing the need for accurate representation with practical constraints such as cost and ethical considerations. Data generated during preclinical studies must be robust, reproducible, and statistically significant. This data will form the foundation of the Investigational New Drug (IND) application, which is required before human clinical trials can commence. These studies need to go beyond simply demonstrating that the therapy "works" in the animal model. They must also provide a detailed understanding of the mechanism of action, potential adverse effects, and the optimal dosage and delivery method. Understanding how the therapy interacts with the body at a cellular and molecular level is crucial for predicting its behavior in humans and mitigating potential risks.

Once preclinical data supports the safety and potential efficacy of the therapy, the next step is filing an IND application with the appropriate regulatory agency. This is a complex and time-consuming process, requiring extensive documentation of all aspects of the therapy's development, from its manufacturing process to the preclinical data supporting its use. The IND application must demonstrate that the proposed clinical trial is ethically sound, scientifically valid, and poses minimal risk to participants. The regulatory agency will carefully review the IND application, and may request additional information or modifications before granting permission to proceed with clinical trials. This review process can take several months, or even years, depending on the complexity of the therapy and the regulatory agency's workload.

Clinical trials are typically conducted in three phases, each with a specific purpose. Phase 1 trials focus on safety and tolerability in a small group of healthy volunteers or patients. The primary goal is to determine the maximum tolerated dose and identify any potential side effects. Phase 2 trials evaluate the efficacy of the therapy in a larger group of patients with the target condition. This phase also continues to assess safety and identify optimal dosing regimens. Phase 3 trials are large, randomized, controlled studies that compare the new therapy to the current standard of care. These trials are designed to definitively demonstrate the efficacy and safety of the therapy in a real-world setting. Each phase of clinical trials requires careful planning, execution, and data analysis. The study protocol must be rigorously adhered to, and patient data must be collected and analyzed in a standardized and unbiased manner. Statistical analysis is crucial for determining whether the observed effects are statistically significant and not simply due to chance.

Another significant hurdle is the manufacturing process. Scaling up production from the laboratory to commercial scale can be a major challenge, particularly for cell-based therapies or complex biomaterials. The manufacturing process must be robust, reproducible, and compliant with Good Manufacturing Practices (GMP). GMP ensures that the therapy is consistently produced to a high standard of quality and purity. Establishing a GMP-compliant manufacturing facility can be a significant investment, requiring specialized equipment, trained personnel, and rigorous quality control procedures. Furthermore, the manufacturing process must be scalable to meet the demands of clinical trials and, eventually, commercial production. This requires careful consideration of factors such as raw material sourcing, process optimization, and automation.

Ethical considerations are also paramount throughout the clinical translation process. Tissue regrowth therapies often involve the use of cells or tissues derived from human donors, raising ethical concerns about informed consent, privacy, and the potential for exploitation. Clinical trials must be conducted in accordance with ethical guidelines, such as the Declaration of Helsinki, and must be approved by an Institutional Review Board (IRB). IRBs are responsible for ensuring that clinical trials are ethically sound and protect the rights and welfare of participants. Patients must be fully informed about the risks and benefits of participating in a clinical trial, and must provide their voluntary informed consent. Furthermore, measures must be taken to protect the privacy of patient data and ensure that it is used only for research purposes. The potential for commercial exploitation of human tissues and cells must also be carefully considered.

Navigating the regulatory landscape is another significant challenge. Regulations governing tissue regrowth therapies vary widely from country to country, and can be complex and constantly evolving. Companies developing these therapies must stay abreast of these regulations and ensure that they are compliant with all applicable requirements. This may involve hiring regulatory consultants or establishing an in-house regulatory affairs department. Failure to comply with regulations can result in delays in approval, or even rejection of the therapy altogether. Securing reimbursement for tissue regrowth therapies can be a major challenge, particularly given their high cost. Payers, such as insurance companies and government healthcare programs, will typically only reimburse for therapies that have been proven to be safe, effective, and cost-effective. Demonstrating cost-effectiveness often requires conducting health economic studies that compare the cost of the new therapy to the cost of existing treatments.

Finally, effective communication is vital throughout the clinical translation process. This includes communication with regulatory agencies, clinical investigators, patients, and the public. Transparency and open communication can build trust and facilitate the development and adoption of new therapies. Clearly communicating the risks and benefits of tissue regrowth therapies is essential for ensuring that patients make informed decisions about their treatment options. Communicating the scientific rationale behind these therapies to the public can also help to build support for research and development efforts. The field of tissue regrowth holds tremendous promise for improving human health. By carefully navigating the challenges of clinical translation, we can bring these innovative therapies to the patients who need them most.

www.ingramcontent.com/pod-product-compliance
Lightning Source LLC
LaVergne TN
LVHW022010200926
848481LV00007B/2316